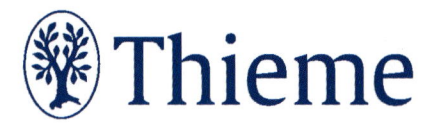

Step-By-Step Approach to Endoscopic Cadaveric Dissection

Paranasal Sinuses and the Ventral Skull Base

Editor-in-Chief

Narayanan Janakiram, MS, DLO
Managing Director
Royal Pearl Hospital
Tiruchirapalli
Tamil Nadu, India

Associate Editors

Dharambir S. Sethi, FRCS (Ed), FAMS (ORL)
Adjunct Associate Professor
Duke–NUS Medical School
Senior Consultant
Novena ENT–Head and Neck Surgery Specialist Centre
Singapore

Onkar K. Deshmukh, MS
Director
Asian Centre for Ear, Nose, and Throat
Indore
Madhya Pradesh, India

Arvindh K. Gananathan
Assistant Surgeon
Vijaya Health Centre
Vijaya Group of Hospitals
Chennai
Tamil Nadu, India

Thieme
Delhi • Stuttgart • New York • Rio de Janeiro

Publishing Director: Dr Sonu Singh
Director-Editorial Services: Rachna Sinha
Project Manager: Gaurav Prabhu
Production Editor: Rohit Bharadwaj
Vice President Sales and Marketing: Arun Kumar Majji
Managing Director & CEO: Ajit Kohli

Copyright © 2019 Thieme Medical and Scientific Publishers Private Limited.

Thieme Medical and Scientific Publishers Private Limited.
A - 12, Second Floor, Sector - 2, Noida - 201 301, Uttar Pradesh, India, +911204556600
Email: customerservice@thieme.in
www.thieme.in

Cover design: Thieme Publishing Group
Typesetting by RECTO Graphics, India

Printed in India by Nutech Print Services

5 4 3 2 1

ISBN: 978-93-88257-06-0
eISBN: 978-93-88257-07-7

Important note: Medicine is an ever-changing science undergoing continual development. Research and clinical experience are continually expanding our knowledge, in particular, our knowledge of proper treatment and drug therapy. Insofar as this book mentions any dosage or application, readers may rest assured that the authors, editors, and publishers have made every effort to ensure that such references are in accordance with **the state of knowledge at the time of production of the book.**

Nevertheless, this does not involve, imply, or express any guarantee or responsibility on the part of the publishers in respect to any dosage instructions and forms of applications stated in the book. **Every user is requested to examine carefully** the manufacturers' leaflets accompanying each drug and to check, if necessary, in consultation with a physician or specialist, whether the dosage schedules mentioned therein or the contraindications stated by the manufacturers differ from the statements made in the present book. Such examination is particularly important with drugs that are either rarely used or have been newly released in the market. Every dosage schedule or every form of application used is entirely at the user's own risk and responsibility. The authors and publishers request every user to report to the publishers any discrepancies or inaccuracies noticed. If errors in this work are found after publication, errata will be posted at www.thieme.com on the product description page.

Some of the product names, patents, and registered designs referred to in this book are in fact registered trademarks or proprietary names even though specific reference to this fact is not always made in the text. Therefore, the appearance of a name without designation as proprietary is not to be construed as a representation by the publisher that it is in the public domain.

This book, including all parts thereof, is legally protected by copyright. Any use, exploitation, or commercialization outside the narrow limits set by copyright legislation without the publisher's consent is illegal and liable to prosecution. This applies in particular to photostat reproduction, copying, mimeographing or duplication of any kind, translating, preparation of microfilms, and electronic data processing and storage.

I dedicate this book to two distinguished people in my life.

My student, Shilpee Bhatia Sharma, who has been in my team for almost all the four-handed procedures performed.

My son, Sathya Narayanan J D, for his ever-growing eagerness to learn that continues to inspire me.

Contents

Foreword   ix
Roman Bošnjak

Foreword   xi
Iype Cherian

Preface   xiii

Contributors   xv

01. Introduction   1
    Narayanan Janakiram

02. Instrumentation for Endoscopic Ventral Skull Base Dissection   7
    Narayanan Janakiram

03. The 15 Commandments in Endonasal Endoscopic Surgery   15
    Narayanan Janakiram

04. Endoscopic Dissection of the Paranasal Sinuses in Functional Endoscopic Sinus Surgery   35
    Narayanan Janakiram, Dharambir S. Sethi, Abhilasha Karunasagar, and Bhanu Pratap Chander

05. Tips and Tricks in Ventral Skull Base Dissection   73
    Narayanan Janakiram, Dharambir S. Sethi, Onkar K. Deshmukh, and Arvindh K. Gananathan

06. Dissection of Vascularized Pedicled Flaps in Ventral Skull Base Reconstruction   83
    Narayanan Janakiram, Dharambir S. Sethi, Onkar K. Deshmukh, and Arvindh K. Gananathan

07. Endoscopic Approaches in Sagittal Plane   105
    Narayanan Janakiram, Dharambir S. Sethi, Arvindh K. Gananathan, and Onkar K. Deshmukh

08. Endoscopic Approaches in Coronal Plane   155
    Narayanan Janakiram, Dharambir S. Sethi, Onkar K. Deshmukh, and Arvindh K. Gananathan

Videos

(1) Middle meatal antrostomy 47

(2) Frontal recess dissection 53

(3) Anterior and posterior ethmoidectomy, sphenoidotomy, and skull base dissection ... 56

(4) Endoscopic DCR—our technique 66

(5) Hadad flap 87

(6) Inferior turbinate flap (lateral nasal wall flap) 92

(7) Transfrontal approach (DRAF III) and endoscopic transnasal craniectomy approach (ACFR) 111

(8) Anatomy of the sphenoid 122

(9) Endoscopic transnasal transsphenoidal approach (endoscopic approach to ventral skull base) 128

(10) Transplanar, trans-sellar, and transtubercular approach 133

(11) Transclival approach 141

(12) Pituitary transposition 142

(13) Optic nerve and orbital decompression 158

(14) Endoscopic endonasal transmaxillary approach (endoscopic modified Denker's procedure and approach to pterygopalatine fossa) 168

(15) Transpterygoid approach to cavernous sinus and approach to infratemporal fossa 177

To view these videos on your smart phone, please download a QR code reader application for your phone. Next, scan the QR codes listed above, and also given on each video image within the chapters. You will get direct access to the videos. To view the videos on your computer, you can access them through the links mentioned at their respective locations in the chapters.

Foreword

Dr Narayanan Janakiram has introduced his dissection manual, *Step-By-Step Approach to Endoscopic Cadaveric Dissection: Paranasal Sinuses and the Ventral Skull Base*, in the era where endoscope-assisted microsurgery is at the zenith of neurosurgical procedures. With modern camera systems and navigation technology, our perception of anatomical structures has dramatically changed and endoscopic anatomy is now established as a novel entity. I have known Dr Janakiram as an excellent surgeon and a passionate teacher, delivering his knowledge across continents, and thereby enabling young minds toward endoscope-assisted surgery. This book is a genuine representation of his passion and skills. It encompasses endoscopic approaches to paranasal sinuses, ventral skull base, cranial nerves, and intracranial space. The readers find themselves in an exclusive area at the crossroads of rhinosurgery and neurosurgery, amalgamated into a unique subspecialty known as endoscopic skull base surgery.

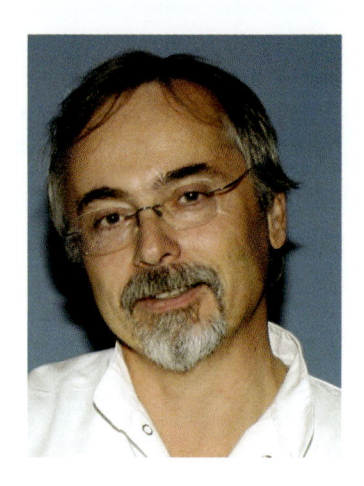

This book is well organized into logical sequence of chapters. First, it deals with instrumentation and basic procedures, leading to complex skull base approaches, which are dealt with in later chapters. The simplicity and power of his 15 commandments enables surgeons to deal with intraoperative challenges. I believe these commandments must be habituated right in their learning phase.

Endoscopic dissection of paranasal sinuses always interests neurosurgeons. This also helps in harvesting various intranasal vascularized pedicled flaps for reconstruction. Tips and tricks of endoscopic ventral skull base dissection are best illustrated by two words—wide exposure. Bi-nostril four-handed approach enables bimanual dissection, which is one of the most effective principles of microsurgery. The essentials of endoscopic approaches in sagittal and coronal planes follow next. These are illustrated by graphical images and photographs.

Although I am more familiar with the sagittal approaches and enthusiastic about cavernous sinus dissection, I read infratemporal fossa, transpterygoid, and petrous approaches with utmost interest and endurance. Here, I realized Dr Janakiram's compassion for propagation of endoscopic skull base surgery.

This book addresses the entire spectrum of expertise—unexperienced and experienced, ENTs and neurosurgeons performing ventral skull base surgery.

Dr Janakiram positions his knowledge and experience from his difficult and extended skull base cases into cadaveric dissection lessons. The most important takeaway message conveyed by this approach is that even experienced surgeons as well as authors cannot dodge the hard work required in the dissection lab.

Endoscope-assisted microsurgery, though minimalistic, is invasive and risky. This book teaches us to follow the principles step-by-step, from paranasal sinuses to skull bases, ascending in complexity from least to the most difficult areas. A must-have book for all skull base surgeons of today and tomorrow.

Roman Bošnjak, MD, PhD
Chief of Department of Neurosurgery
University Medical Centre Ljubljana;
President of Slovenian Neurosurgical Society;
President of Neuroendoscopy Committee of South-east
European Neurosurgical Society (SeENS)
Ljubljana, Slovenia

Foreword

For years, the teaching and learning in neurosurgery has faced several stumbling blocks with respect to the integration of advancement and improvement of techniques in it with the progress of time. The valuable experience gained by surgeons with years of success, failures, and hard work was not passed on to the next generation of surgeons because of attitude issues, poor teaching material, and an absence of smooth integration of the will to learn and the passion to teach.

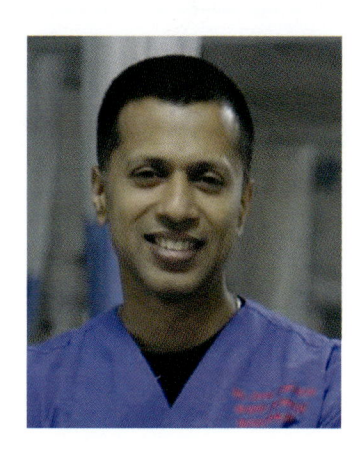

In this book, Narayanan Janakiram takes us through his years of hard work, reaching new heights of excellence in endoscopic skull base surgery. His experience has been poured out in the most elegant way possible, something only he can do in his inimitable style.

This book would be a valuable asset for beginners as well as expert neurosurgeons, embarking on the difficult journey of endoscopic skull base surgery. I would like to congratulate Narayanan on this stupendous effort and encourage readers to strive to learn more from this book.

Iype Cherian
Director and Chair
Nobel Institute of Neurosciences
Nobel Medical College and Teaching Hospital
Biratnagar, Nepal

Preface

As a resident, during my tenure in Madras Medical College, I had the privilege of being mentored by great teachers like Prof G. Gananathan and Prof M. K. Rajashekar, who were a constant source of inspiration to me. My training in endoscopic sinus surgery was undertaken under the able tutelage of renowned surgeons such as Prof D. S. Sethi and Prof P. J. Wormald, who strengthened my foundation in sinus surgery and thus paved the way for me to become a skull base surgeon.

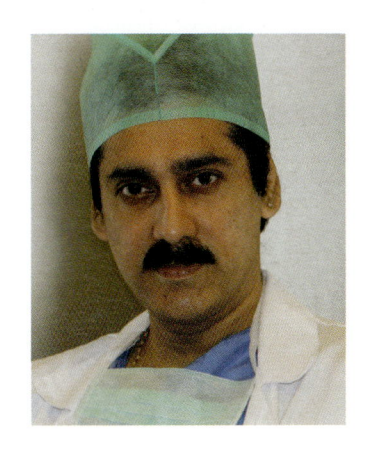

Watching eminent surgeons like Prof Amin Kassam and Prof Ricardo Carrau invoked in me a profound interest in the field of skull base surgery and inspired me to write my first book *Navigation of Sinuses and Ventral Skull Base—Comprehensive Approach to Basic and Advanced Techniques with Radiological Correlations*. An in-depth knowledge in skull base surgery facilitated me to develop new concepts on a very sinister tumor—juvenile nasopharyngeal angiofibroma, which once again gave me the confidence to write another book—*Juvenile Nasopharyngeal Angiofibroma*. The substantial success of these two books motivated me to write this book—*Step-by-Step Approach to Endoscopic Cadaveric Dissection: Paranasal Sinuses and the Ventral Skull Base*.

Skull base surgery is an ever-evolving discipline. Advances in the past two decades have significantly altered the way we approach lesions of the ventral skull base. Cadaveric dissections form an essential element in the training of a skull base surgeon to foster the necessary skills that would enable one to operate with ease and dexterity. I advise all aspiring skull base surgeons (neurosurgeons and ENT surgeons) to perform as many cadaveric dissections as possible in order to shorten the steep learning curve involved in performing complex surgical procedures.

Skull base surgery is an art as well as a science and every young surgeon must attempt to enhance their skills by performing structured and meticulous cadaveric dissections. This endeavor to perfect one's skills and achieve expertise is a life-long journey and a goal that every skull base surgeon must strive to accomplish.

I conclude with a small piece of advice to youngsters. I request you to respect all your teachers who have taught you not only to perform advanced surgeries, but also those who taught you the basics such as technique of holding an endoscope. Their blessings will make you a complete surgeon and a refined human being.

I hope this book will provide the younger generation of aspiring surgeons with the required knowledge of the basic concepts for performing cadaveric dissections, thus, empowering them to achieve excellence in skull base surgery.

Narayanan Janakiram

Contributors

Abhilasha Karunasagar, MS (ENT)
Junior Consultant
Royal Pearl Hospital
Tiruchirapalli
Tamil Nadu, India

Bhanu Pratap Chander, MS (ENT)
Junior Consultant
Royal Pearl Hospital
Tiruchirapalli
Tamil Nadu, India

01 Introduction

Narayanan Janakiram

The modern-day endonasal endoscopic surgery is a culmination of the dynamic interplay between advances in medicine, technology, and growing surgical expertise. The endonasal endoscopic corridor is now the preferred approach for diseases of the nose and paranasal sinuses. Nonetheless, the endonasal corridor has also emerged as a primary route to access almost all pathologies along the ventral skull base.

Before the emergence of the endoscopic route, the patients with nasal ailments often endured significant morbidity and cosmetic blemish from open approaches. Attempts for nasal endoscopy were made since 1901, but the actual impetus for endoscopic sinus surgery was provided by the creation of the Hopkins rod lens system in the 1960s. In the following decade, functional endoscopic sinus surgery evolved from the pioneering works of Messerklinger, Wigand, and other researchers. Thereafter, the popularity of functional endoscopic sinus surgery quickly escalated to encompass indications beyond inflammatory pathologies.

The evolution of endonasal skull-base surgery is as interesting as the surgery itself. Though the first report of transsphenoidal resection of pituitary tumor was described in 1907 by Henry Schoffer, this approach represents a combination of century-long developments in fields of neurosurgery, neuroanatomy, pathology, and technology. Harvey Cushing initially adopted this route for skull-base lesions, but later gave it up in favor of transcranial route. However, it was the conviction of contemporaries like Norman Dott, Gerard Guiot, and Jules Hardy who facilitated the resurgence of this route. Around the same time, the development of the rod lens telescope and consequent development in rhinology paved the way for the development of endonasal endoscopic approaches.

In the past few decades, this approach has been transformed from an optional alternative to an essential workhorse corridor for ventral skull-base surgery. This metamorphosis can be credited to innumerable contributions made by neurosurgeons and rhinologists all around the globe; ventral skull-base pathologies from the frontal lobe to the clivus and further down to atlantoaxial joint and those extending up to infratemporal fossa and cavernous sinus laterally are now routinely accessed via these corridors. These approaches have the distinctive advantages of being cosmetically superior, having deeper access and better tumor clearance, reduced complications, and postoperative hospital stay and thereby better surgical outcomes.

As fascinating as it may seem, endonasal endoscopic surgery in some instances can prove to be a daunting task. Loss of depth perception due to a two-dimensional image, anatomical and topographical disorientation due to a faulty camera angle, and fogging of the telescopic lens due to blood and secretions can cause visuospatial disturbances. Owing to restricted maneuverability and erroneous judgement of the instruments in limited endonasal space, surgeons sometimes struggle to translate their movements in to effective surgical steps. This may result in undesired tissue trauma and sometimes even perilous complications. Furthermore, nonergonomic posturing and grips especially in the learning phase can result in considerable surgical fatigue.

Though a myriad of articles describes various endonasal endoscopic techniques in great details, those on ergonomics in endonasal endoscopy still remain scanty. Based on his extensive experience in endonasal endoscopic sinus and skull-base surgery over the last two decades, the senior author has devised certain principles governing posturing, positioning, and placement of endoscopic instruments. It is to the author's experience and belief that habituating these guidelines would enable a trainee surgeon to negotiate the learning curve, gain surgical confidence, reduce operative time, and make endoscopic surgery comfortable and graceful.

Through this dissection manual, the author endeavors to evoke interest regarding endonasal endoscopic surgery in young eager minds. The following chapters describe in details the basics of endonasal endoscopy, instrumentation, and cadaveric dissection for functional endoscopic sinus surgery and approaches in ventral skull-base surgery. There are numerous high-quality pictures in the manual that are extracted from author's cadaveric dissections. They depict extent of exposures that one should achieve and important structures that one encounters during dissection along these endoscopic approaches. The authors have made a sincere effort to orient the readers with endoscopic anatomy, habituate them to utilize instrument in the most effective manner, and familiarize them with various endonasal endoscopic approaches.

02 Instrumentation for Endoscopic Ventral Skull Base Dissection

Narayanan Janakiram

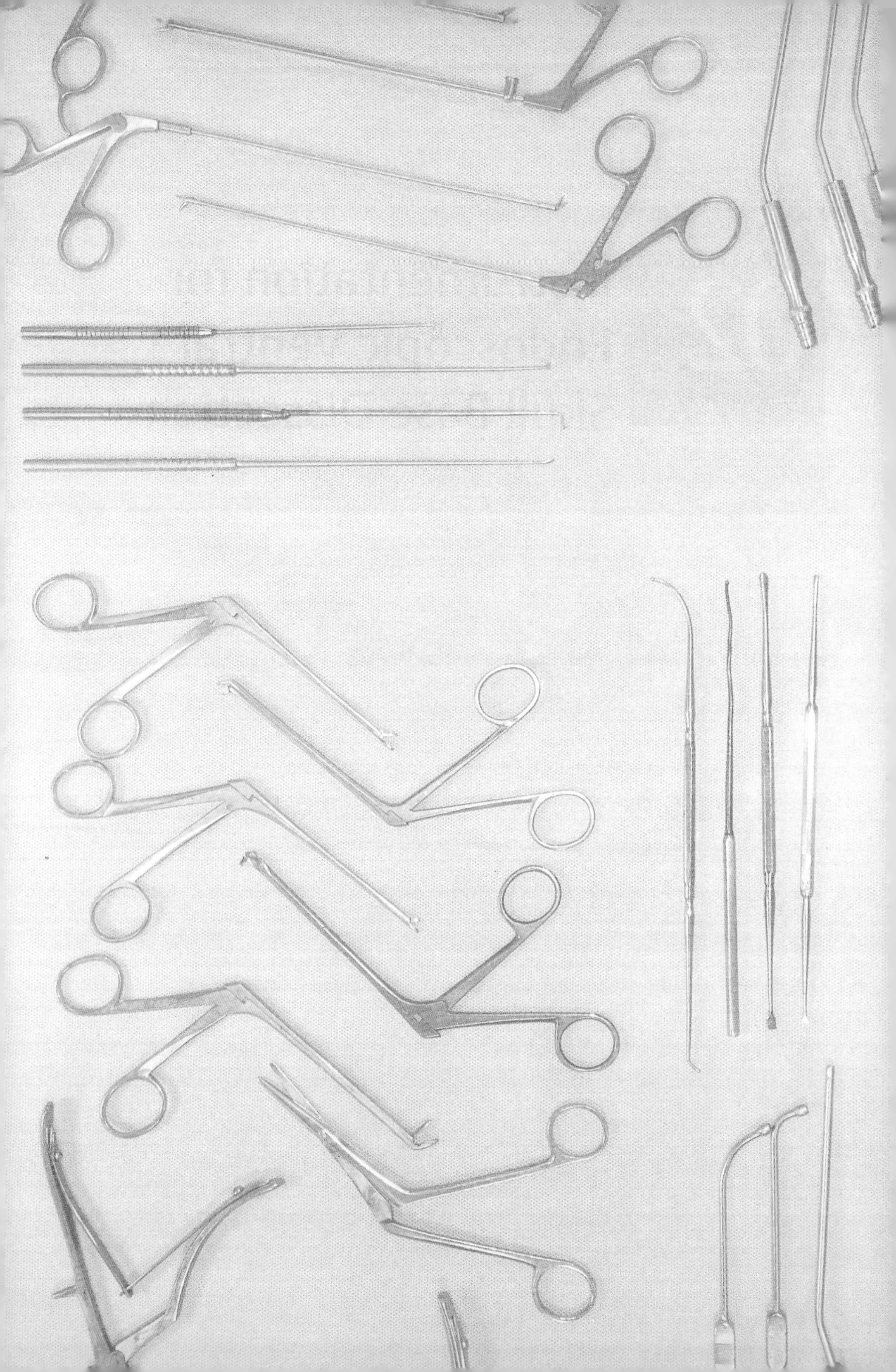

Instrumentation for Endoscopic Ventral Skull Base Dissection

Instrumentation is the medium through which a surgeon expresses his/her knowledge, attitude, and practice toward the subject. Prudent instruments simplify surgeries and make them safe and elegant. Stellar instruments are an essential prerequisite for a modern-day surgery.

Instrumentation is of vital importance in endoscopic skull base surgery. In endoscopic surgeries, surgeons do not have a direct contact with tissues and organs, thereby losing flexibility and tactile feedback. Endoscopic instruments should translate surgeon's movements to the tissues and carry tactile feedbacks from the tissues back to the surgeon, thereby becoming an extension of surgeon's body and thought process.

Endoscopic skull base surgery is a microsurgery dealing with critical neurovascular structures and demands refined movements. A specialized dedicated endoscopic skull base instrument set is a primary prerequisite for any endoscopic skull base surgery and even for skull base dissection.

The authors strongly recommend the use of same instrumentation for endoscopic skull base surgeries as well as cadaveric dissections. This, they believe, will habituate the dissector to use specific instrument for a particular step of the surgery, thereby establishing fixed operative protocols very much during the learning phase itself.

Ventral skull base instrumentation includes an endoscopic camera system (**Figs. 2.1, 2.2**), a set of cold steel instruments (**Fig. 2.3**), powered instruments, hemostatic instruments such as the electrocautery, and the navigation systems. During cadaveric dissections, the authors recommend the dissector to be equipped with camera system with recording facility, a dedicated set of skull base instruments, and powered instruments such as the high-speed drill system and the micro-debrider shaver system.

The high-speed neurodrill systems (**Figs. 2.4, 2.5**) assist the surgeon in effective bone removal with minimal damage to surrounding structures. An experienced surgeon can also estimate parameters such as thickness of the bone, density, and consistency of the underlying tissue from the visual, tactile, and auditory feedback of the drill. It is important to irrigate the high-speed drill burr to avoid heat damage to the tissue and to have a clear visualization of the field.

The shaver system (**Fig. 2.6**) has an important role in functional endoscopic sinus surgery (FESS) and nasal phase of ventral skull base surgery. It is a very efficient tool for mucosa preservation in FESS. The simultaneous debridement of the mucosa (sparing the bone) and suction-irrigation helps to achieve effective removal of mucosal pathology and maintain a clear field. Its primary application in ventral skull base surgery is limited to the nasal phase, where exposures or corridors are created by removal of paranasal sinuses.

The following is a set of instruments used by the authors while performing his dissection.

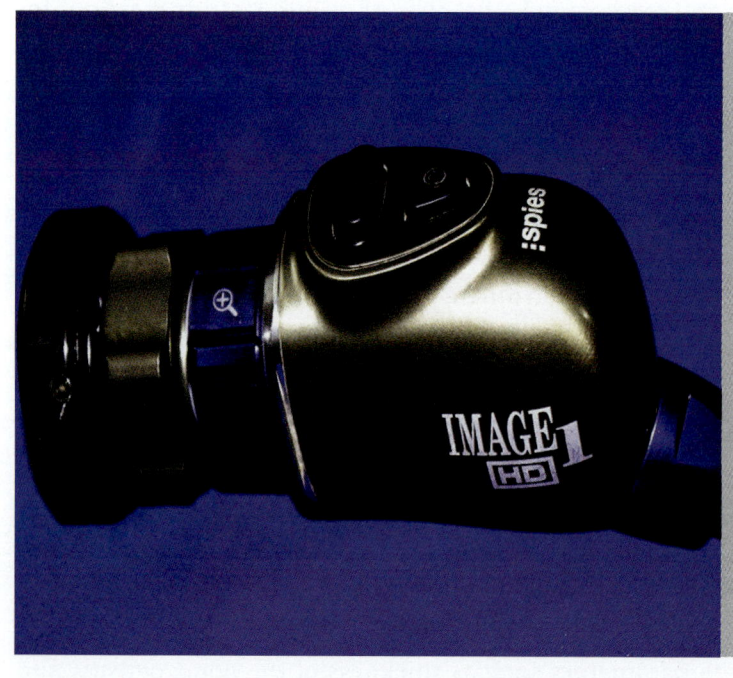

Fig. 2.1 Camera head of an endoscopic system used for dissection.

Instrumentation for Endoscopic Ventral Skull Base Dissection

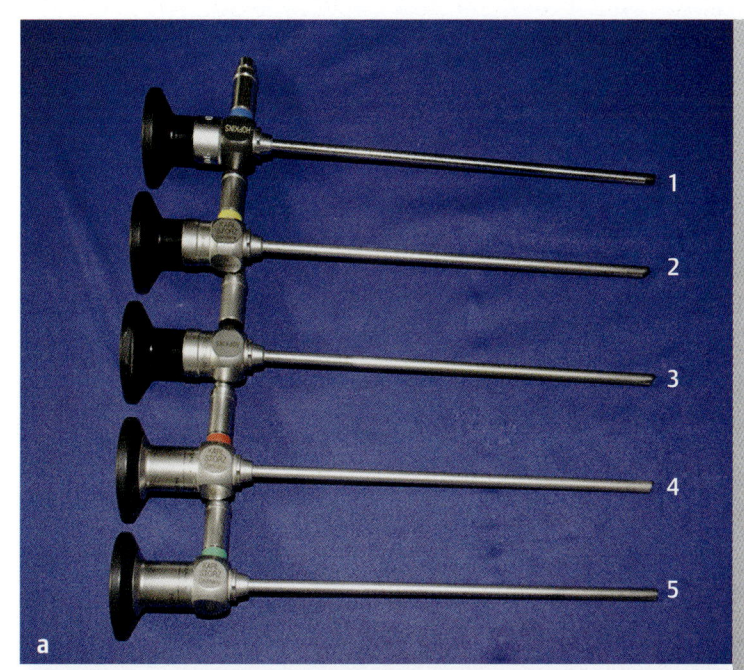

Fig. 2.2 **(a, b)** Various endoscopes used in ventral skull base dissection. (1–5 depict the different angled views they provide including 0, 30, 45, 70, and 90 degrees.)

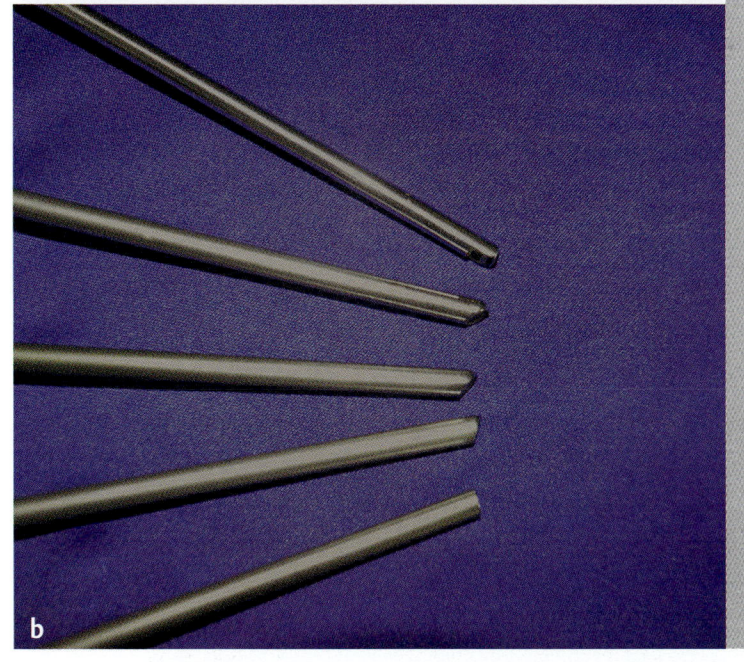

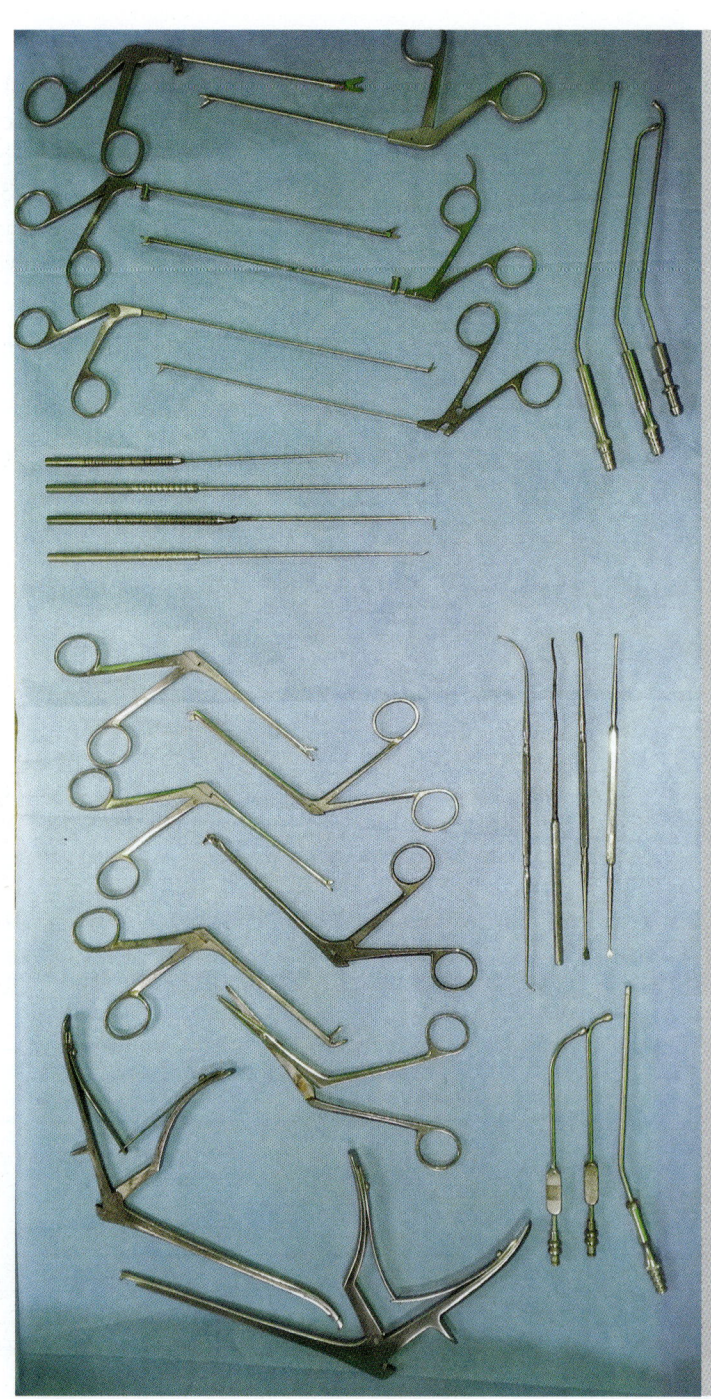

Fig. 2.3 Set of instruments dedicated for functional endoscopic sinus surgery and ventral skull base surgery.

Instrumentation for Endoscopic Ventral Skull Base Dissection 13

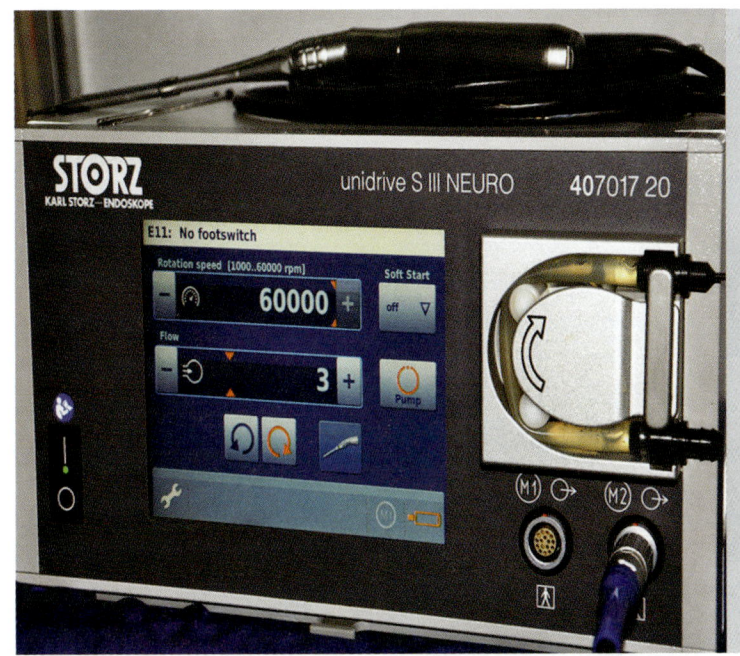

Fig. 2.4 High-speed neurodrill system.

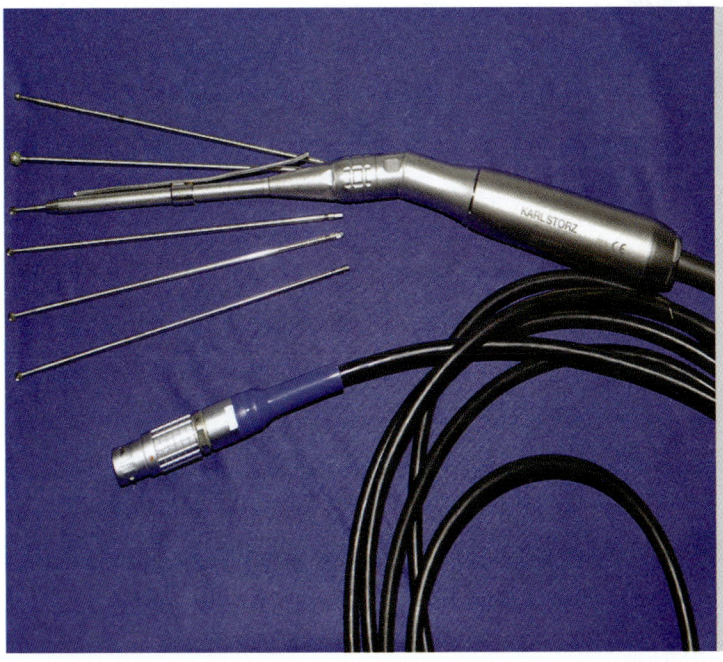

Fig. 2.5 Contra-angled handpiece of the drill provides ergonomic and effective bone removal.

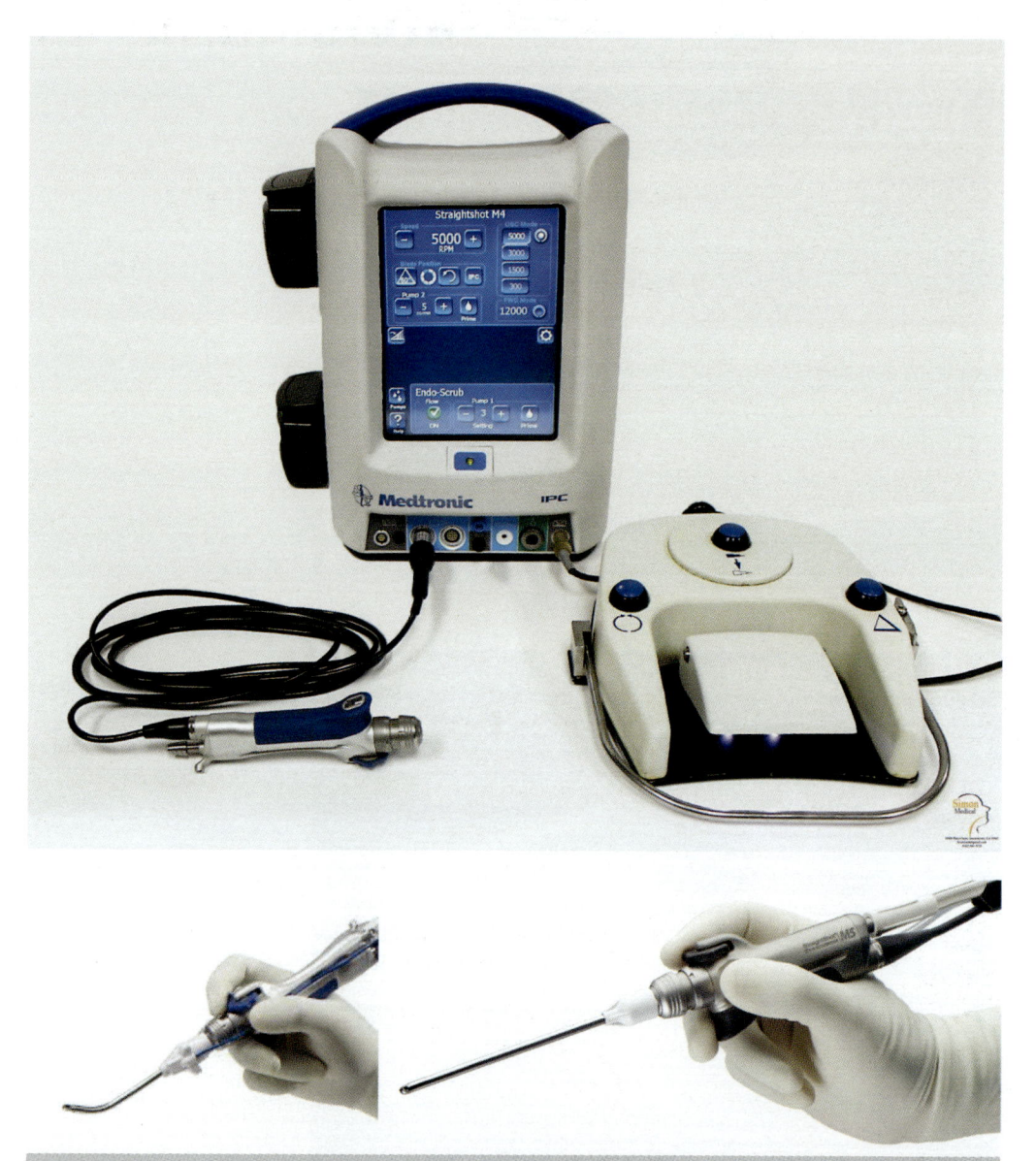

Fig. 2.6 Micro-debrider/shaver system with straight and angled blade.

03 The 15 Commandments in Endonasal Endoscopic Surgery

Narayanan Janakiram

- § How to Get Started with Endoscopic Surgery 17
- § Commandment 1 17
- § Commandment 2 19
- § Commandment 3 20
- § Commandment 4 20
- § Commandment 5 23
- § Commandment 6 23
- § Commandment 7 24
- § Commandment 8 25
- § Commandment 9 28
- § Commandment 10 29
- § Commandment 11 29
- § Commandment 12 29
- § Commandment 13 30
- § Commandment 14 31
- § Commandment 15 32
- § Conclusion 33

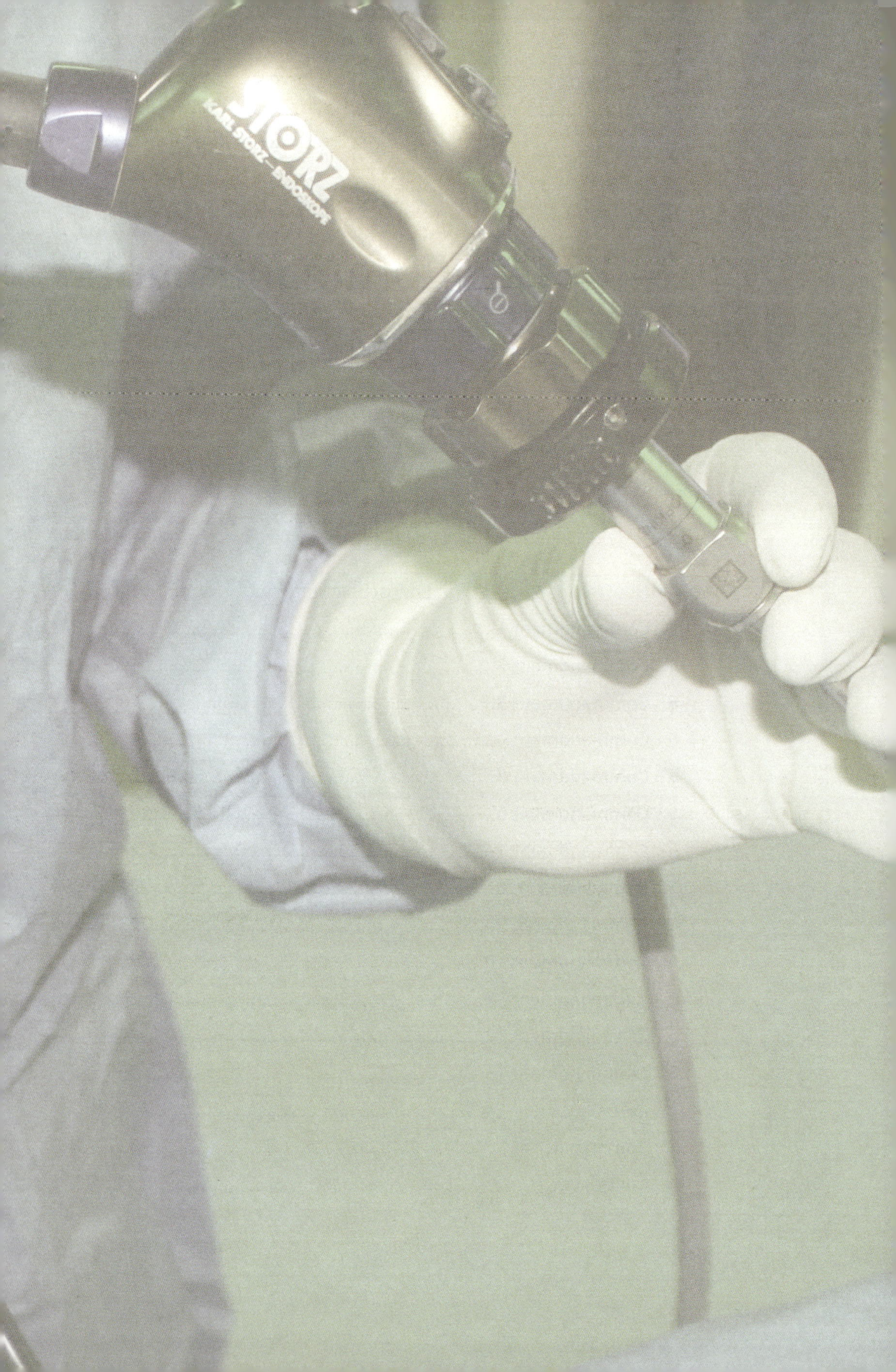
STORZ
KARL STORZ—ENDOSKOPE

The 15 Commandments in Endonasal Endoscopic Surgery

How to Get Started with Endoscopic Surgery

Mastering the functional endoscopic sinus surgery and skull base surgery has a long learning curve. From a neurosurgical point of view, the new skillset is required working off a two-dimensional image than the three-dimensional image. Proper training in endoscope and instrument handling with hand-eye coordination is required to avoid unnecessary morbidity and mortality.

This section of the book deals with the bare basic steps involved in starting off with endoscopic sinus surgery.

Commandment 1

Position of the Patient

During the endoscopic procedures, reverse Trendelenburg's position is preferred with the head in neutral position (**Fig. 3.1**). A slight tilt of the patient's head toward the surgeon is preferred.

To keep the head in flexed position is recommended for beginners doing functional endoscopic sinus surgery (FESS) as it is difficult to reach the skull base, but it has the disadvantage of not reaching the frontal sinus. This position can be achieved by placing a sandbag under the patient's occiput so that the neck is flexed (**Fig. 3.2**). The extended head position is recommended for doing the frontal sinus surgery. This position can be achieved by placing the sandbag under the patient's neck so that the head gets extended (**Fig. 3.3**). The most preferred position of the head will be in neutral position, and the 0-degree telescope is in line with the floor of the nasal cavity.

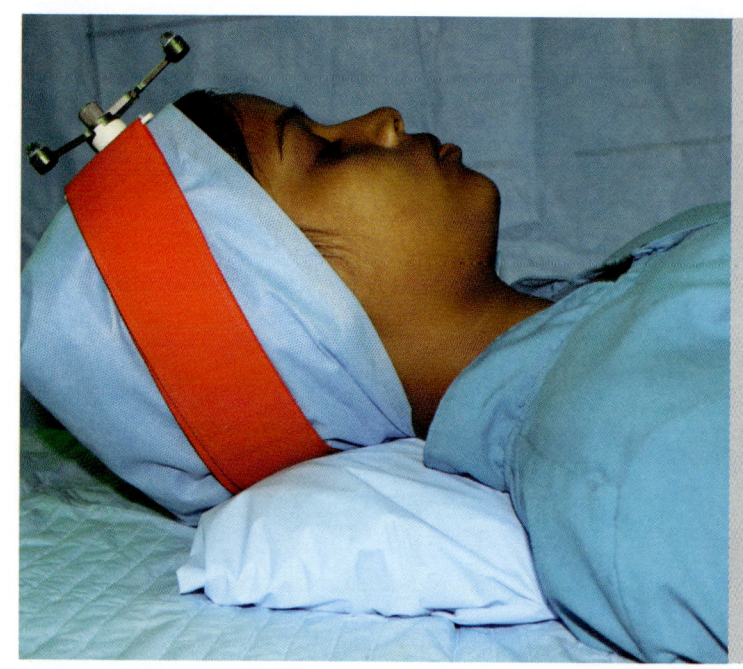

Fig. 3.1 Patient's head in neutral position.

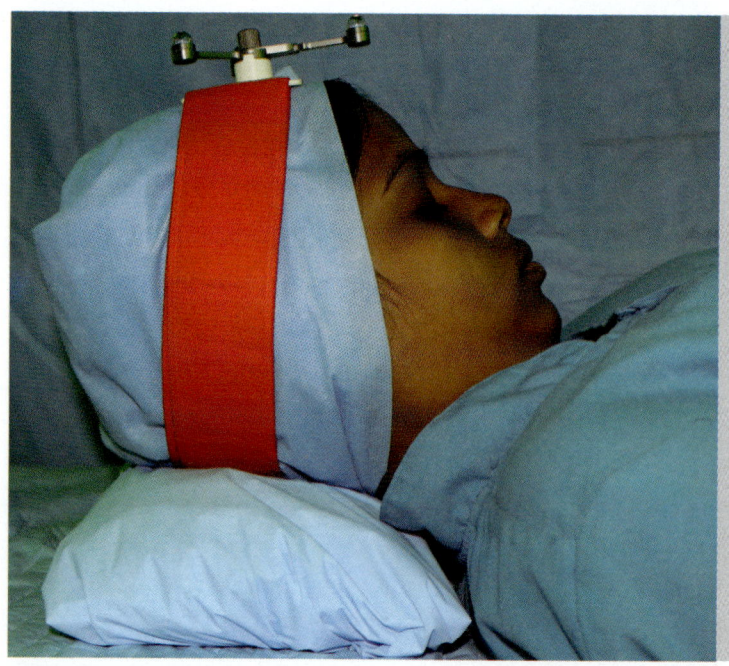

Fig. 3.2 Patient's head in flexed position.

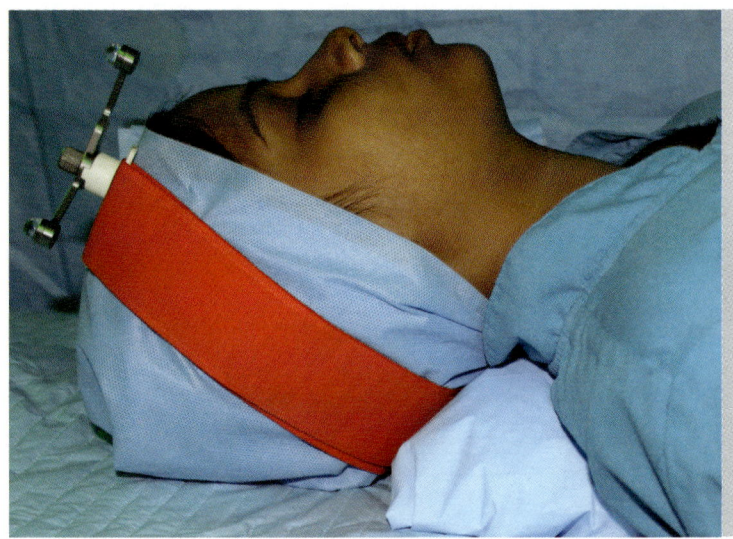

The 15 Commandments in Endonasal Endoscopic Surgery

Fig. 3.3 Patient's head in extended position.

Commandment 2

The scope should be held like a flute as depicted in **Fig. 3.4**. It is not advisable to hold the camera.

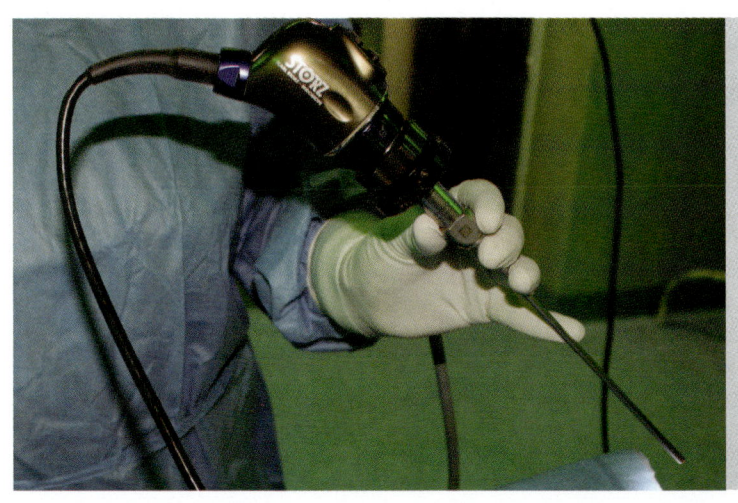

Fig. 3.4 Holding of the endoscope.

Commandment 3

It is preferable to keep the cable of the camera and the light source to the left of the patient to decrease the weight of the cables (**Fig. 3.5**).

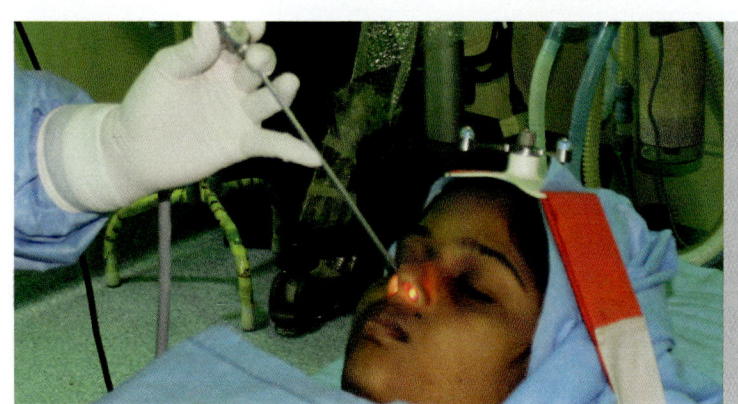

Fig. 3.5 The cables of camera and light source hanging over the left side of the patient.

Commandment 4

The scope is introduced by taking advantage of the elasticity of the alar cartilage (**Fig. 3.6**).

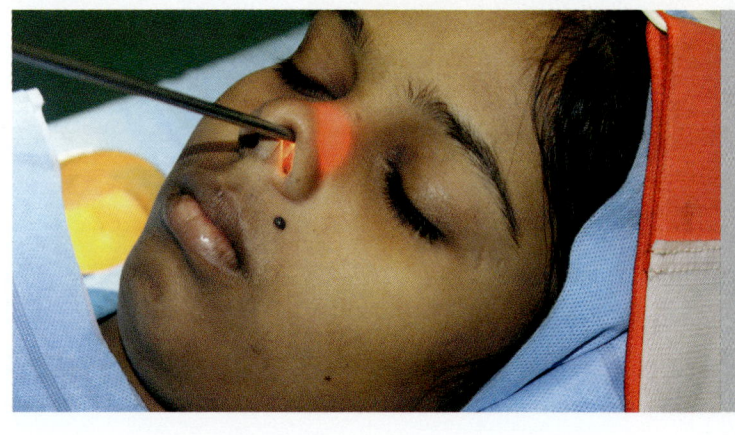

Fig. 3.6 Introduction of the scope by using the alar elasticity.

The Semilunar Sign

On introduction of the 0-degree telescope, impingement on any structure in the nasal cavity will produce a crescentic rim of light along a portion of the circumference of the endo picture. This is called the "semilunar sign." This indicates that the scope should be moved 180 degrees away from its current position (**Figs. 3.7, 3.8**). This helps avoid injury to the structure and fogging of the telescope leading to the reduction in operating time.

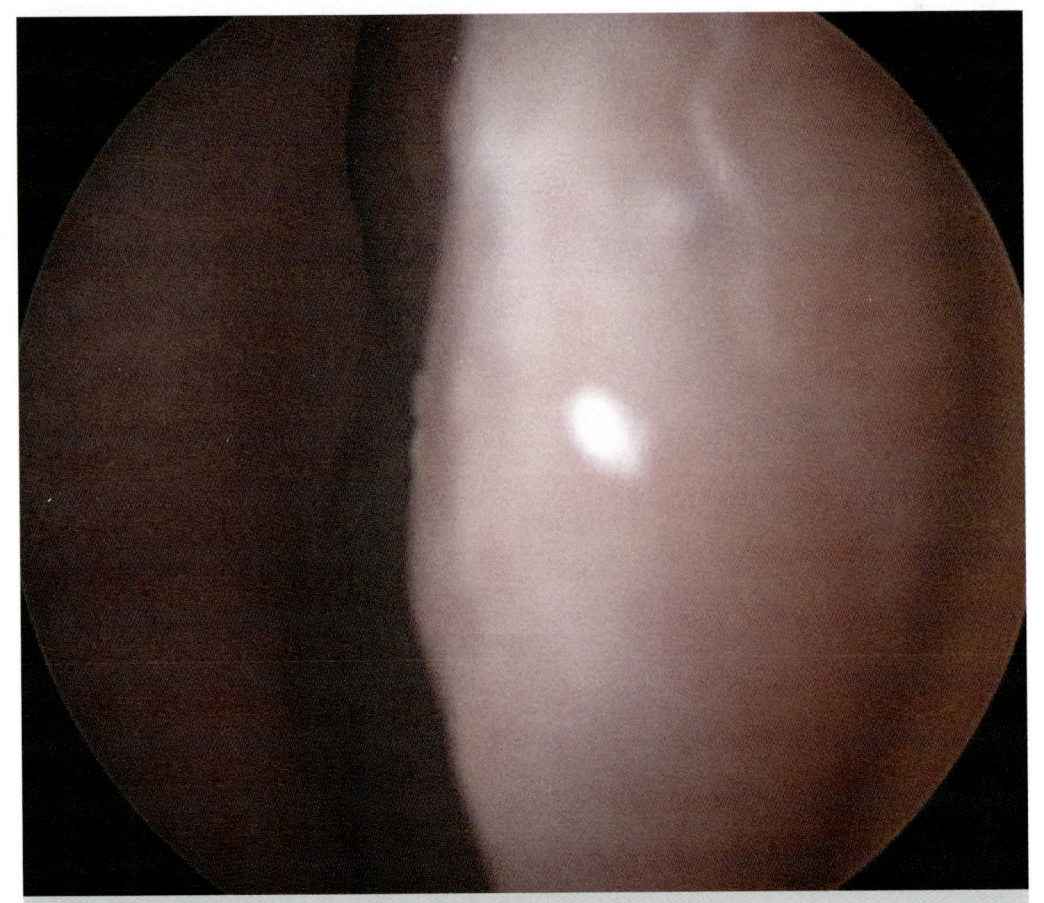

Fig. 3.7 Semilunar sign.

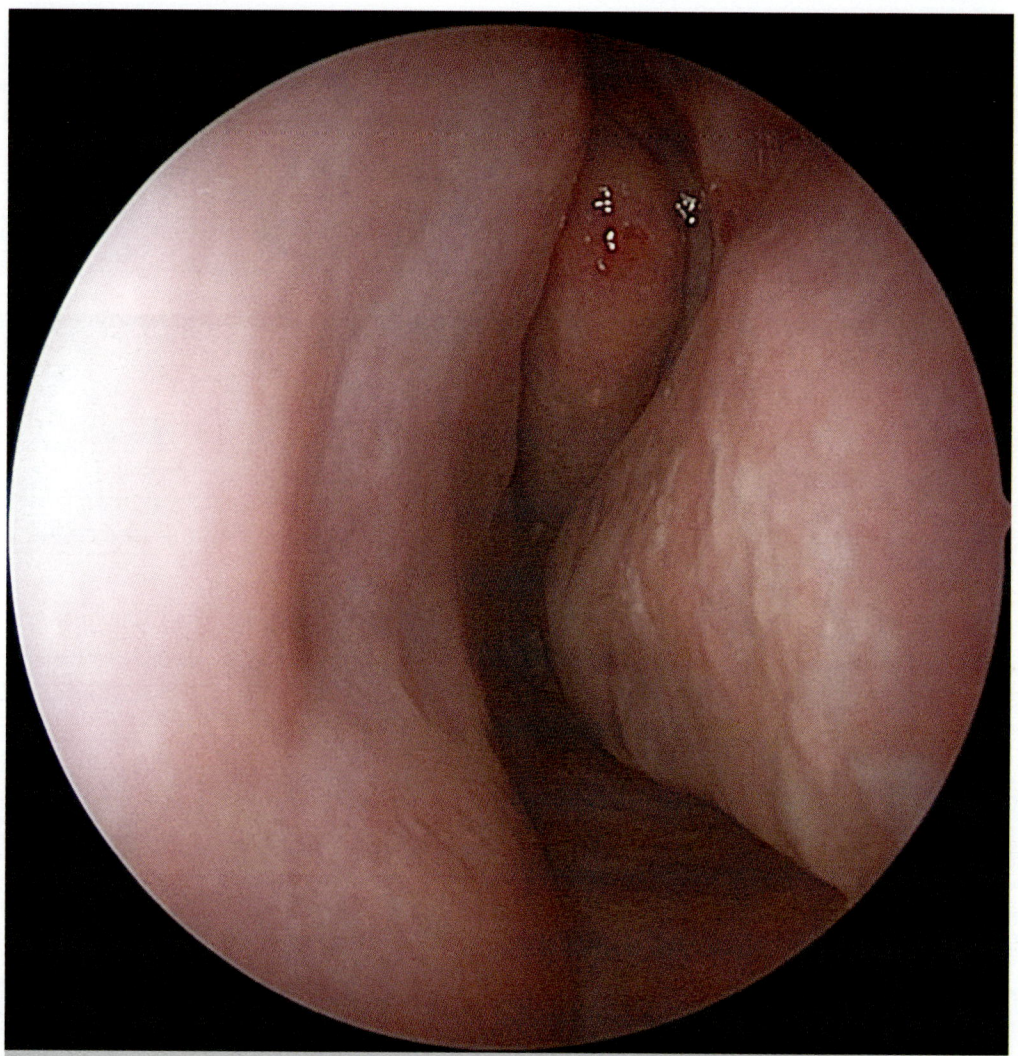

Fig. 3.8 Scope moved away 180 degrees to get the correct view.

Commandment 5

The instrument is introduced utilizing the rigidity of the floor of the nasal cavity (**Fig. 3.9**).

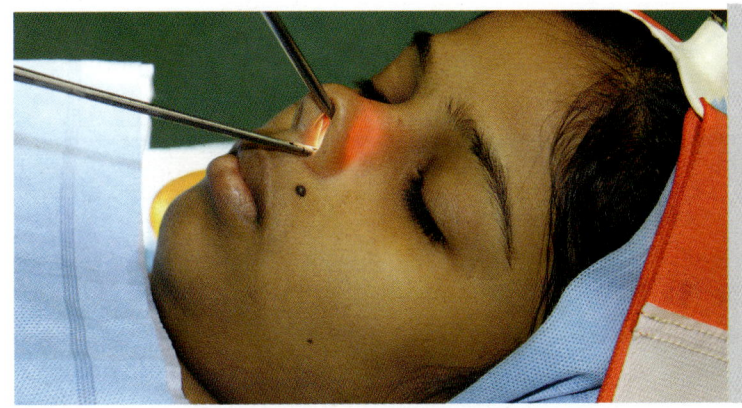

Fig. 3.9 Introduction of the instrument along the floor.

Commandment 6

The crossover should be avoided, and at no point, the instrument and scope should touch each other (**Fig. 3.10**).

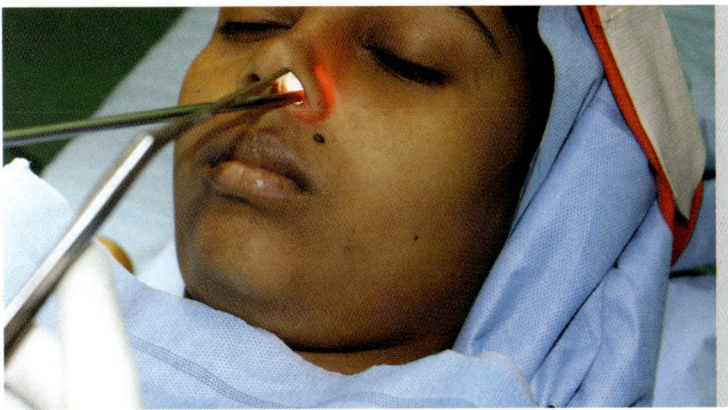

Fig. 3.10 Crossover phenomenon.

Commandment 7

The endoscopic view of the instrument tip should always be maintained while introducing the instruments in the nasal cavity, especially sharp-tipped instruments (**Fig. 3.11**).

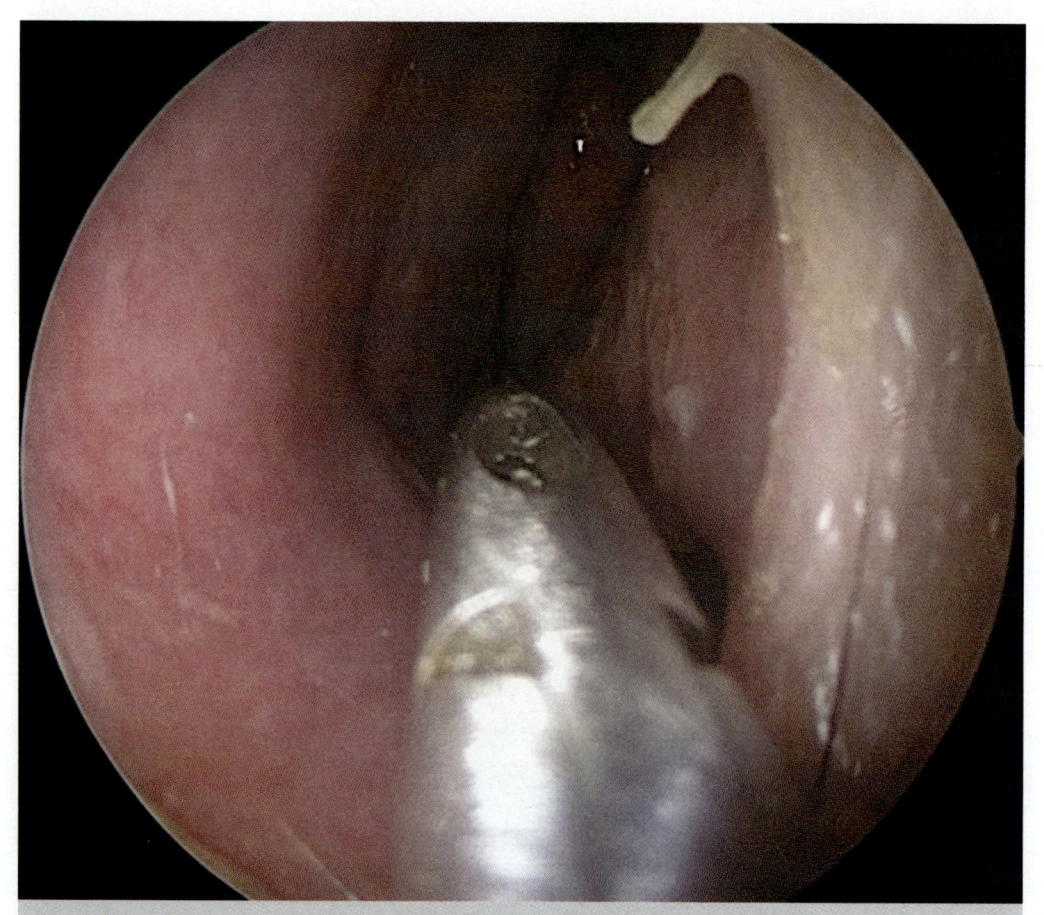

Fig. 3.11 The scope and instrument being advanced simultaneously.

Commandment 8

The distance between the instrument tip and scope tip should always be constant (~1.5–2 cm in FESS and 2.5 cm in endoscopic skull base surgery) (**Figs. 3.12–3.14**). This principle of constant distance may not be applicable in the four-handed technique used for expanded endonasal approaches.

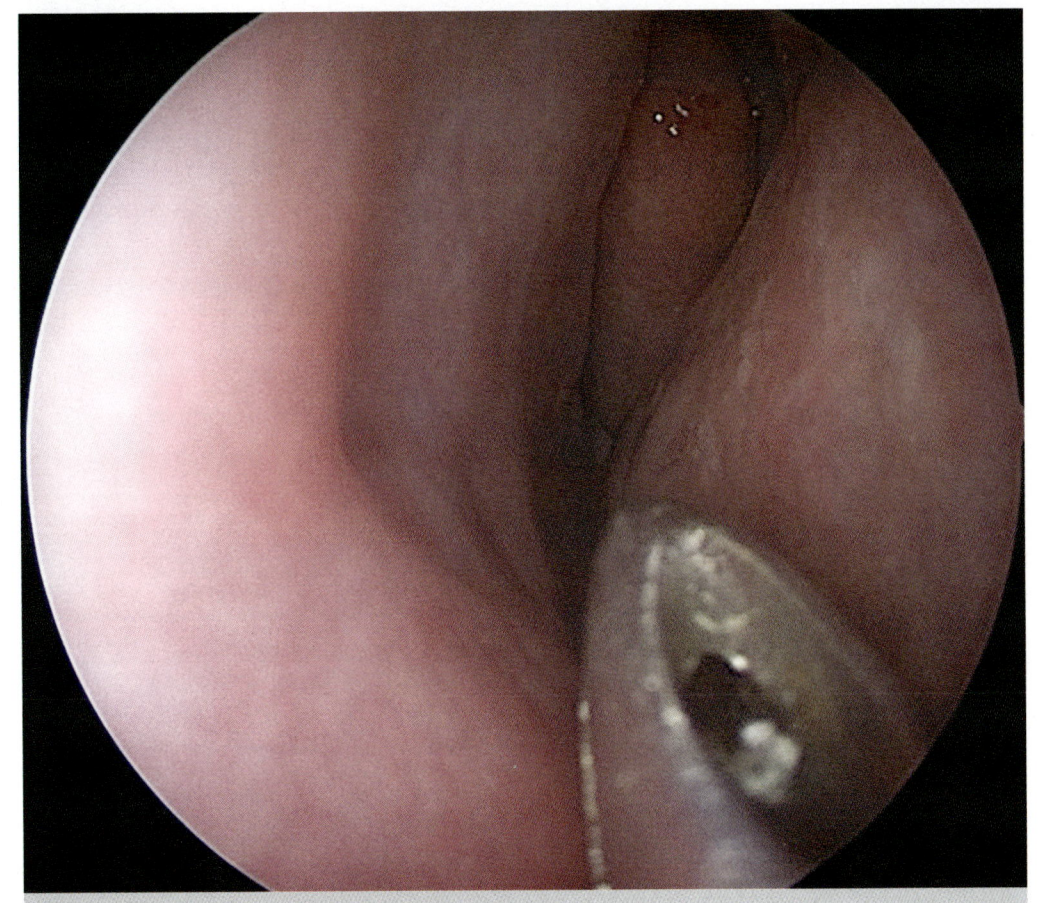

Fig. 3.12   The instrument too close to scope.

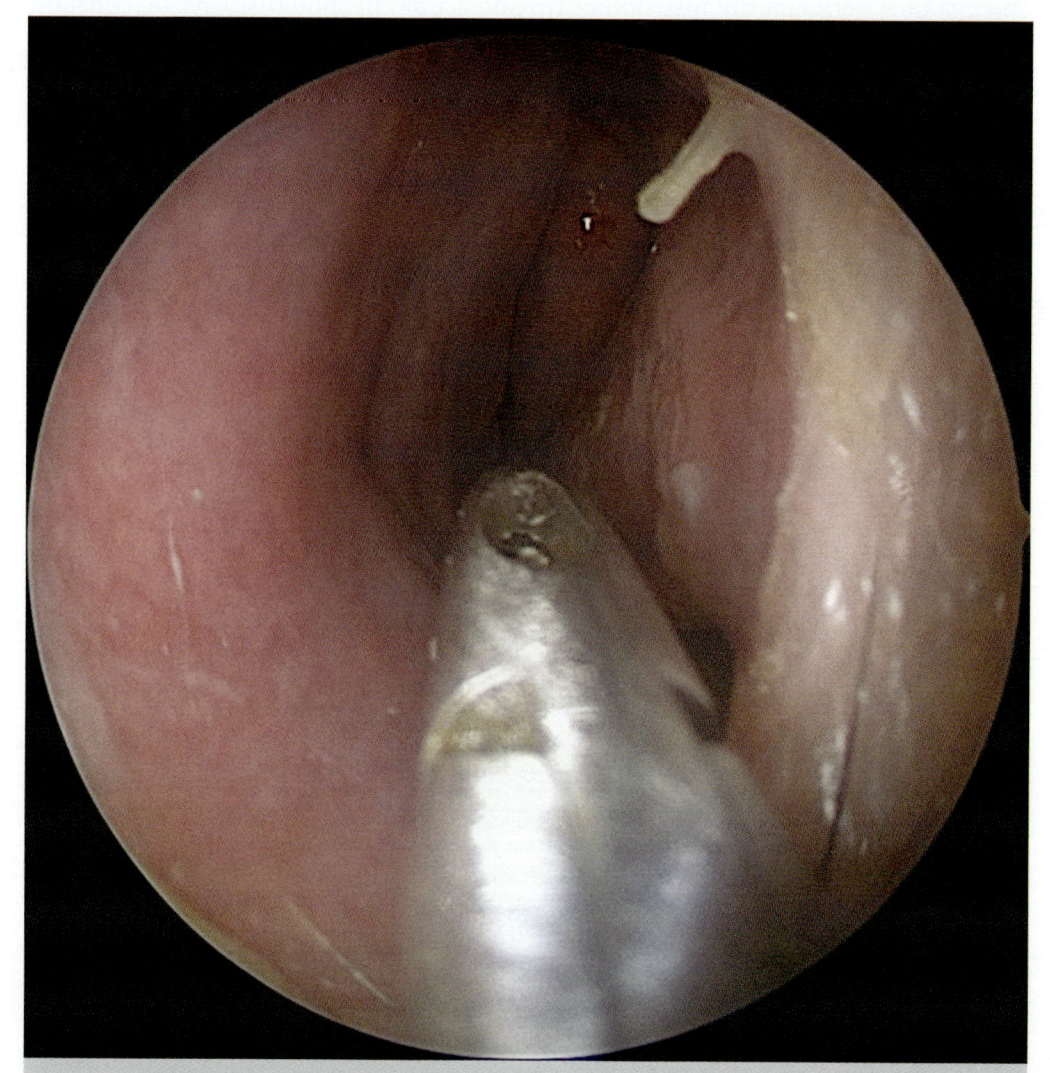

Fig. 3.13 The optimum instrument distance from the scope.

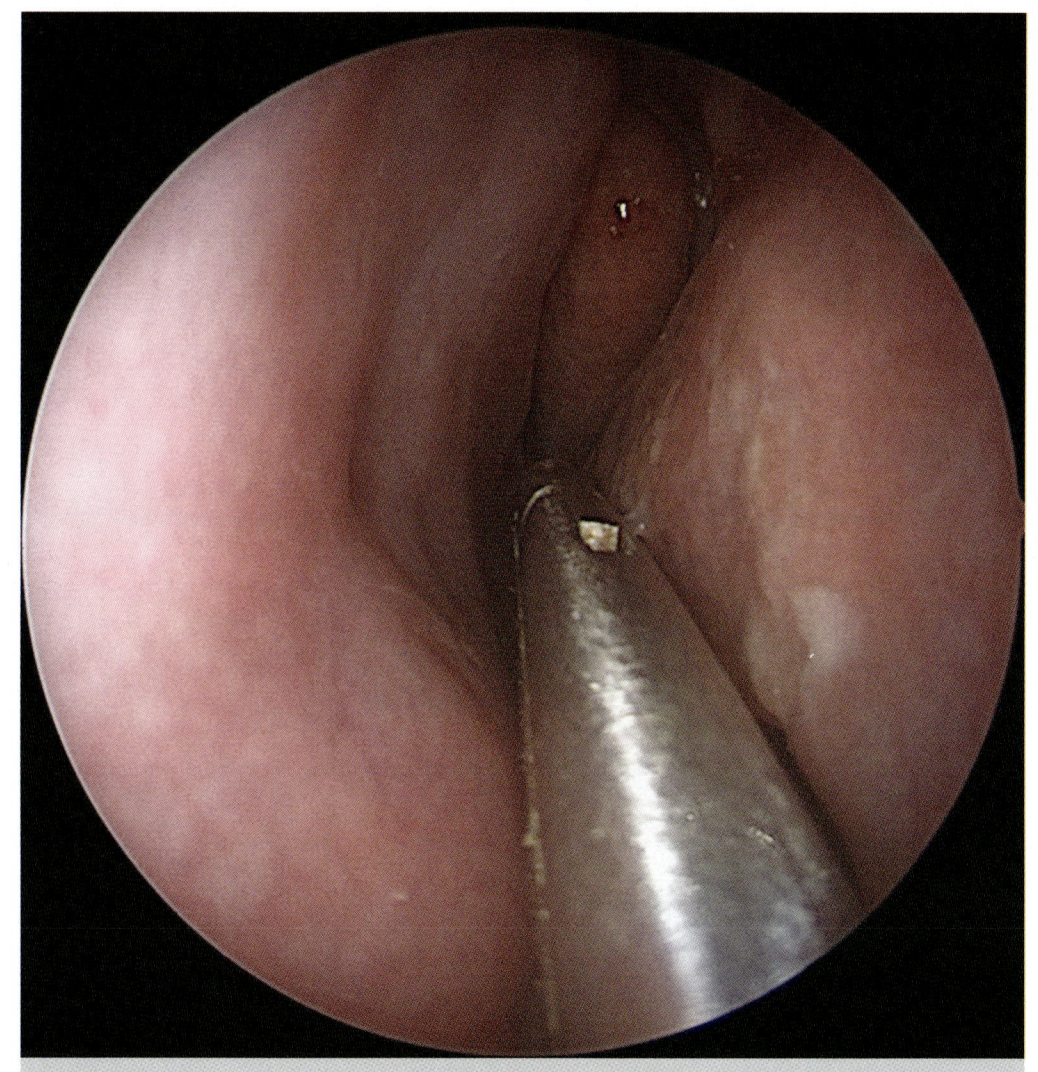

The 15 Commandments in Endonasal Endoscopic Surgery

Fig. 3.14 Instrument too distant from the scope.

Chapter 03

Commandment 9

To facilitate the 0-degree view, angled scopes are introduced into the nasal cavity and moved in an arc to view the part to be operated; 0- and 30-degree telescopes have zero views (**Fig. 3.15**). Hence, this applies to 45-, 70-, and 90-degree telescopes (**Fig. 3.16**).

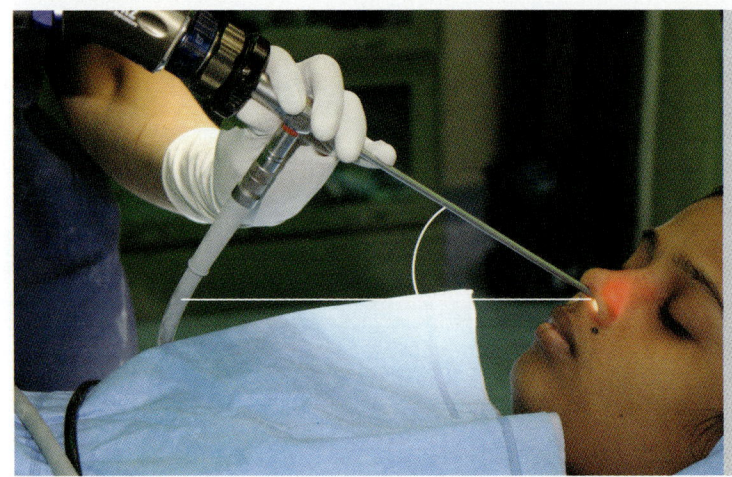

Fig. 3.15 Angle of introduction of 30-degree telescope.

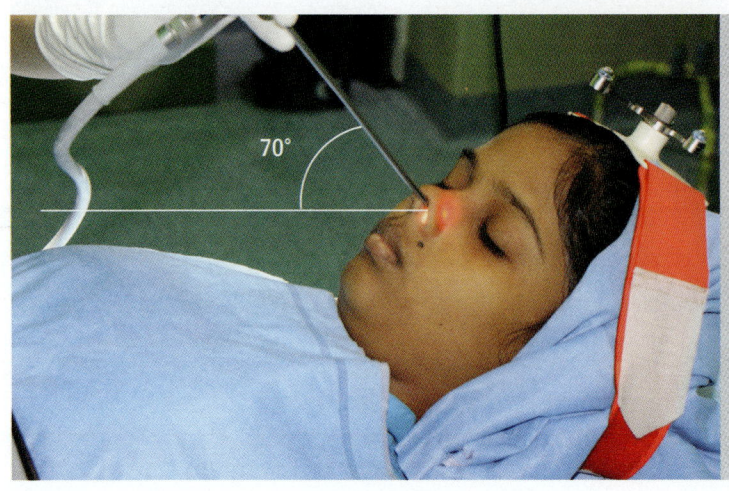

Fig. 3.16 Angle of introduction of 70-degree telescope.

Commandment 10

Have an aerial view of the part being operated, and the scope should give a panoramic view of the area.

Commandment 11

Never pull or pluck tissue unless you see the instrument tip.

Commandment 12

Always use the instrument below the telescope unless you are operating in the frontal recess. During the frontal recess surgery to view the tip, the instrument should have an angle greater than the telescope.

Commandment 13

The hemostatic measures used are adrenaline (1:1,000) soaked lints (well squeezed) or to use saline at the 40°C temperature as this promotes the clotting mechanism (**Fig. 3.17**).

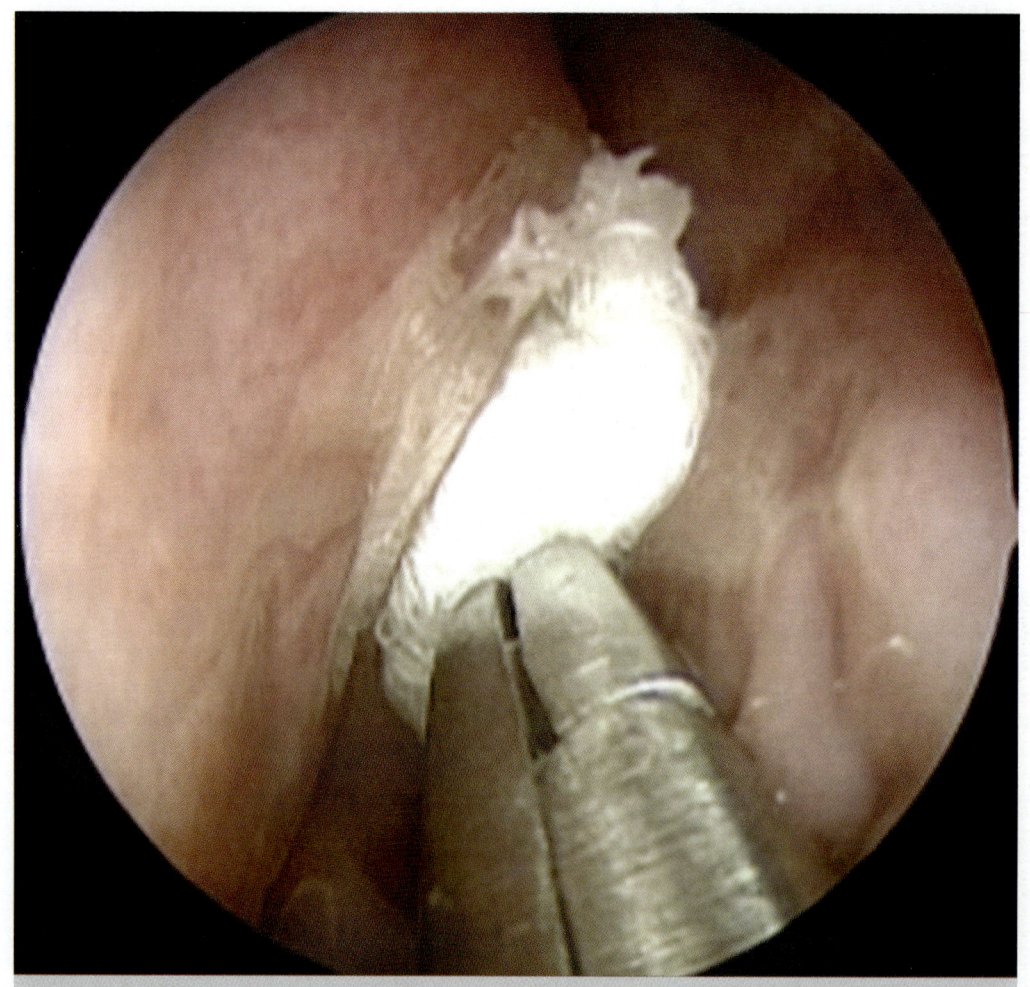

Fig. 3.17 Adrenaline lint used for topical decongestion.

The 15 Commandments in Endonasal Endoscopic Surgery

Commandment 14

Gentle manipulation of the middle turbinate is to be done to prevent the fracture of the turbinate (**Fig. 3.18**). The lesser the scope fogs, the faster you operate.

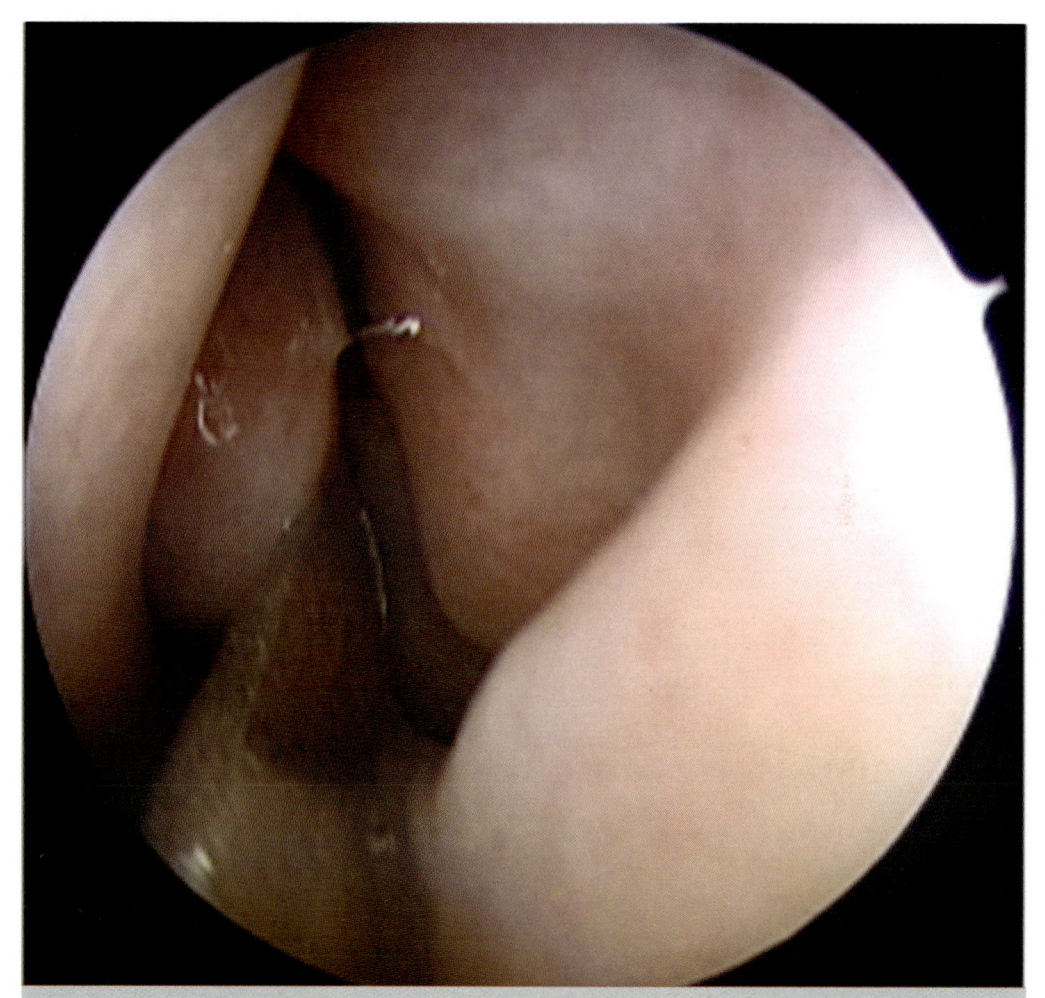

Fig. 3.18 Scope manipulated into the middle meatus by gently pushing the middle turbinate medially.

Chapter 03

Commandment 15

Camera tilt should be avoided as this gives a totally false sense of orientation to prevent the complications (**Fig. 3.19**). The incisor teeth or philtrum can be used as a marker to orient oneself before the introduction of the telescope.

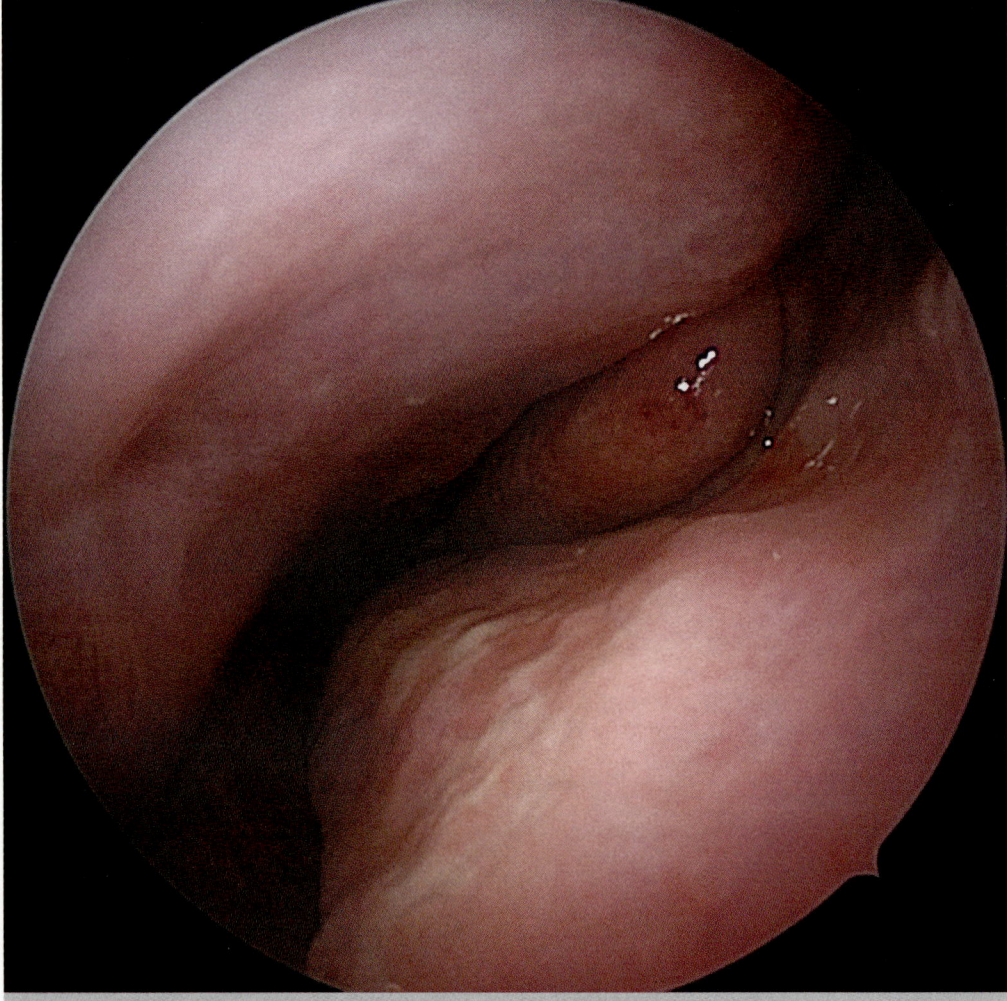

Fig. 3.19 Camera tilt.

Conclusion

Beginners of endoscopic sinus surgery meet with a series of challenges before they achieve finesse and dexterity. In the author's perception, it is not only the knowledge of anatomy but strict adherence to basic principles, right from the handling of the telescope to the proper orientation of the field during surgery, which makes the surgeon shorten the steep learning curve, thus making him/her a perfect surgeon. In view of this, the author has designed the "Jr sinus model" to practice hand-eye coordination before performing surgeries on patients.

NOTE: The 15 commandments have been conceived by the author.

04 Endoscopic Dissection of the Paranasal Sinuses in Functional Endoscopic Sinus Surgery

Narayanan Janakiram, Dharambir S. Sethi, Abhilasha Karunasagar, and Bhanu Pratap Chander

- § Introduction 37
- § Cadaver Dissection for FESS 37
- § Nasal Endoscopy 38
- § Uncinectomy 39
- § Middle Meatal Antrostomy (Video 1) 47
- § The Frontal Sinus Recess 51
- § Frontal Recess Dissection (Video 2) 52
- § Dissection of Anterior Ethmoid (Video 3) 56
- § Dissection of Posterior Ethmoid (Video 3) 59
- § Dissection of Sphenoid Sinus (Video 3) 61
- § Endoscopic Dacryocystorhinostomy— Modified Approach (Video 4) 66

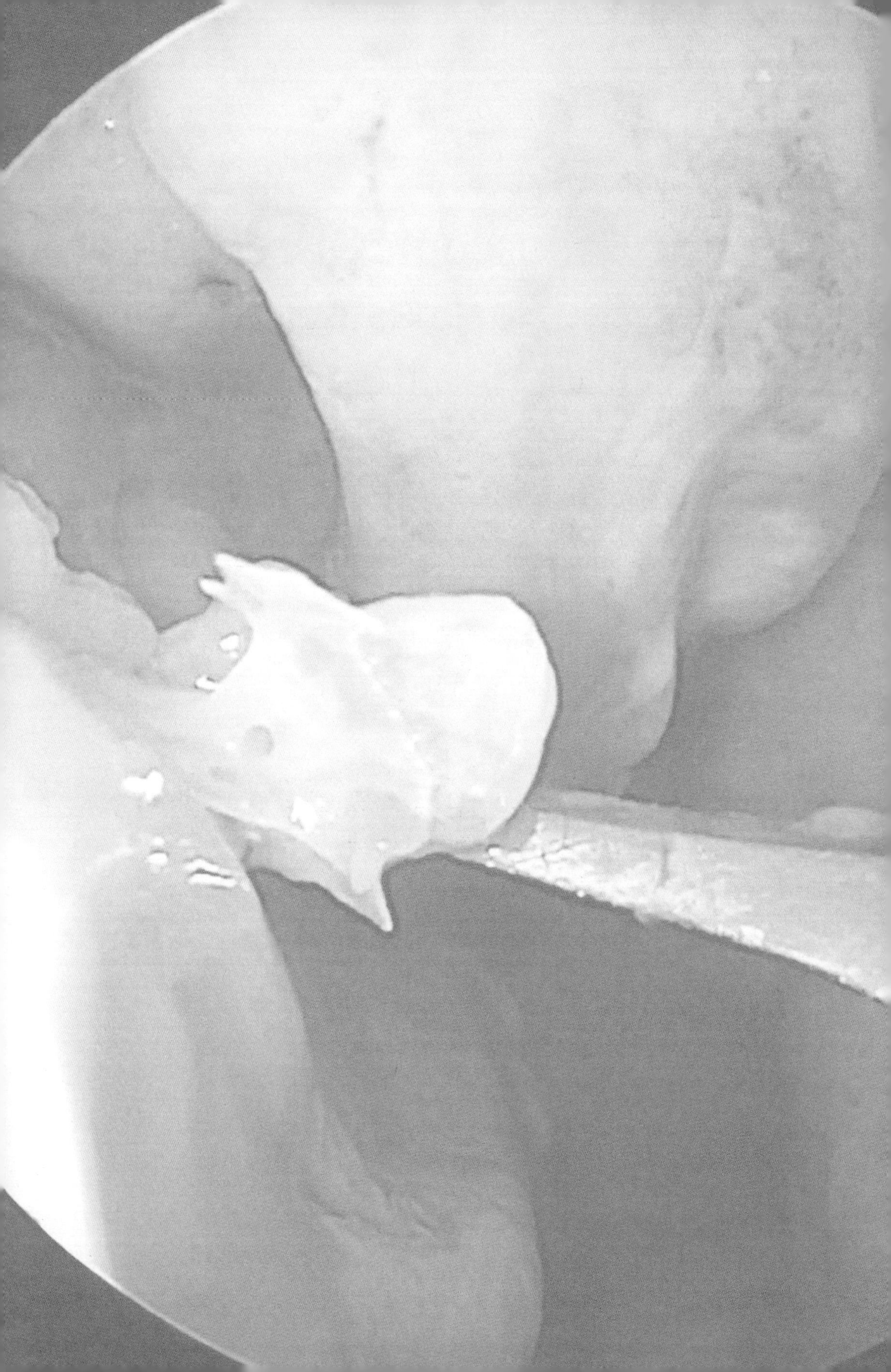

Introduction

Stammberger and Posawetz[1] suggested that the primary inflammatory process commences in the nose and the ethmoid sinuses that secondarily affects the bigger maxillary and frontal sinuses. The disease initially affects an area that is collectively referred to as the osteomeatal complex (OMC). This represents the confluence of drainage pathways for the frontal and maxillary sinuses. The Messerklinger technique aims at removal of the ethmoid air cells and widening the prechambers to the frontal and maxillary sinus at the OMC to re-establish ventilation and drainage. It was observed that functional restoration of sinus physiology could be achieved by addressing the pathology in OMC; widening the ethmoidal infundibulum (prechamber for maxillary sinus) and frontal recess (prechamber for frontal sinus) sufficed to treat inflammatory sinus pathology without any major manipulations in the bigger maxillary and frontal sinuses per say.[1]

Restoration of sinus drainage and ventilation via endonasal endoscopic surgery was referred to as functional endoscopic sinus surgery (FESS) by Kennedy in 1985. This surgery rapidly gained popularity and soon it was the standard approach for the management of inflammatory disease of the nose. Today, the indications for the endonasal endoscopic route have expanded to encompass almost all pathologies of the nose and ventral skull-base. Endoscopic orientation and technique are the primary prerequisites for any endonasal procedures.

Cadaver Dissection for FESS

Cadaver dissections form a vital part of learning and making of a skilled competent surgeon. Anatomical points of interest are similar to that of living tissues in fresh-frozen cadavers in contrast to formalin preserved ones where the tissues lose their pliability. This chapter deals with various exercises in endoscopic sinus surgery with a detailed video description. Although numerous strategies are available to perform a particular step, this chapter describes the methodology as performed by the author.

Nasal Endoscopy

The authors describe here a novel technique of performing office endoscopy called *"The Aircraft technique."*

A 0-degree telescope is introduced utilizing the elasticity of the ala of nose. At the level of anterior end of inferior turbinate, the telescope is angulated such that it "takes off" and "flies" between the middle and inferior turbinate and "lands" in the nasopharynx. The sphenoethmoidal recess is examined as the telescope is withdrawn. Anatomical variations/pathology in any of these areas may have been visioned with a single pass.

Note the following structures; these are important landmarks in primary FESS:

- Inferior turbinate
- Middle turbinate
- Axilla of middle meatus
- Uncinate process; bulla ethmoidalis
- Accessory ostia
- Tubal elevation; Eustachian tube
- Fossa of Rosenmuller
- Superior turbinate; sphenoid os

The Middle Turbinate

The middle turbinate is one of the main landmarks in a case of primary FESS. Every attachment of the MT is of vital importance in endoscopic orientation. The anterior most attachment marks the beginning of the maxillary line and forms the axilla. This is an important landmark in locating the lacrimal sac and the frontal recess. Similarly, the ground lamella demarcates the transition between the anterior and the posterior ethmoidal cell. Sometimes pneumatization of the middle turbinate or a paradoxical curvature may encroach upon the middle meatus and obstruct the osteomeatal unit. During such conditions, it may be lateralized or partially resected but otherwise, the author recommends to retain and preserve the middle turbinate as far as possible in a FESS.

Uncinectomy

The Uncinate Process

The uncinate process is thin, sickle-shaped, and runs almost in the sagittal plane from anterosuperior to posteroinferior. It has a posterior free margin which usually lies parallel to the anterior surface of the ethmoidal bulla.

The uncinate bone has three parts: the horizontal portion, the middle portion, and the superior portion. The horizontal portion is attached to the ethmoidal process of inferior turbinate and palatine bone, the middle portion is attached to the lacrimal bone and lamina papyracea, and the superior portion will extend to a varying degree into the frontal recess, determining the frontal recess drainage.[2]

The uncinate process has three superior attachments: the medial orbital wall, the middle turbinate, and the skull base. However, in some cases, multiple attachments have been noted.[2,3]

According to Landsberg and Friedman, there are six variations in superior attachment of uncinate namely (**Fig. 4.1**):

- **Type 1:** Insertion to the lamina papyracea (52%)
- **Type 2:** Insertion to the posteromedial wall of the agger nasi cell (18.5%)
- **Type 3:** Insertion to both the lamina papyracea and the junction of the middle turbinate with the cribriform plate (17.5%)
- **Type 4:** Insertion to the junction of the middle turbinate with the cribriform plate (7%)
- **Type 5:** Insertion to the skull base (3.6%)
- **Type 6:** Insertion to the middle turbinate (1.4%)[4]

The uncinate attaches to the medial orbital wall in 85% of cases;[3] thus, the frontal sinus drainage is medial to uncinate. In 15% of the cases,[3] uncinate gets attached to the middle turbinate or skull base. In such cases, the frontal recess drains lateral to uncinate process.

The variants of uncinate process include medialized, lateralized, everted (paradoxical), occasionally pneumatized.

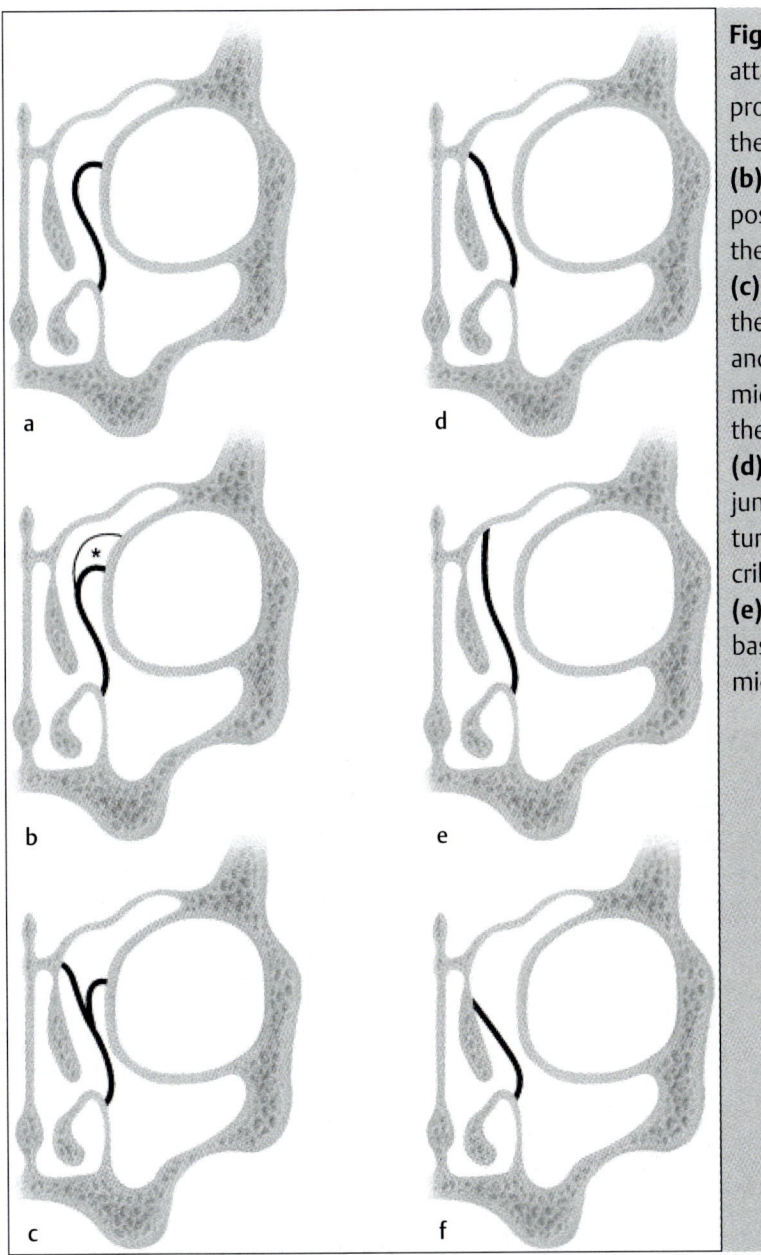

Endoscopic Dissection of the Paranasal Sinuses

Fig. 4.1 Superior attachments of uncinate process. **(a)** Insertion to the lamina papyracea. **(b)** Insertion to the posteromedial wall of the agger nasi cell. **(c)** Insertion to both the lamina papyracea and the junction of the middle turbinate with the cribriform plate. **(d)** Insertion to the junction of the middle turbinate with the cribriform plate. **(e)** Insertion to the skull base. **(f)** Insertion to the middle turbinate.[4]

Dissection

Structures to be identified initially (**Fig. 4.2**):

- Anterior attachment of uncinate to the lacrimal crest
- Free border of uncinate process
- Hiatus semilunaris inferioris—a two-dimensional cleft between the bulla and uncinate process (**Fig. 4.3**)
- Bulla ethmoidalis (**Fig. 4.4**)

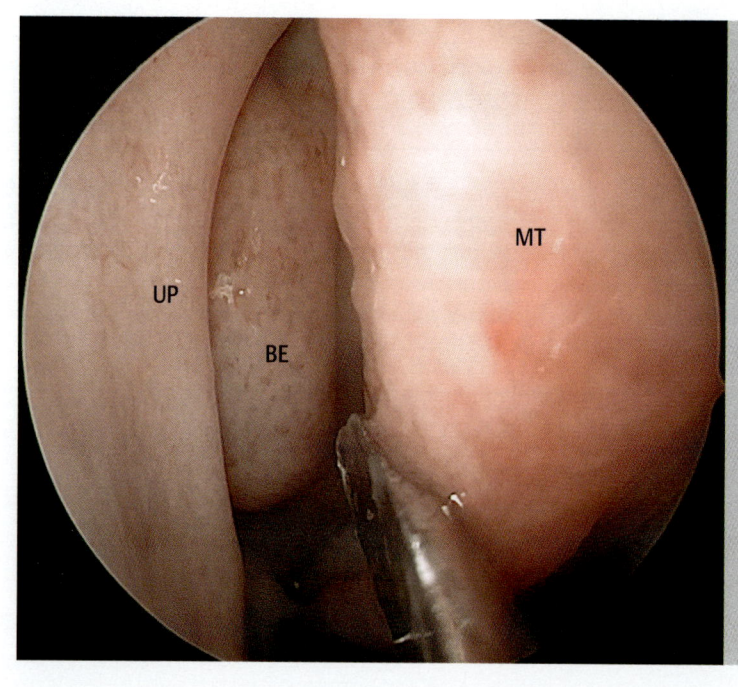

Fig. 4.2 Identifying posterior margin of uncinate process. BE, bulla ethmoidalis; MT, middle turbinate; UP, uncinate process.

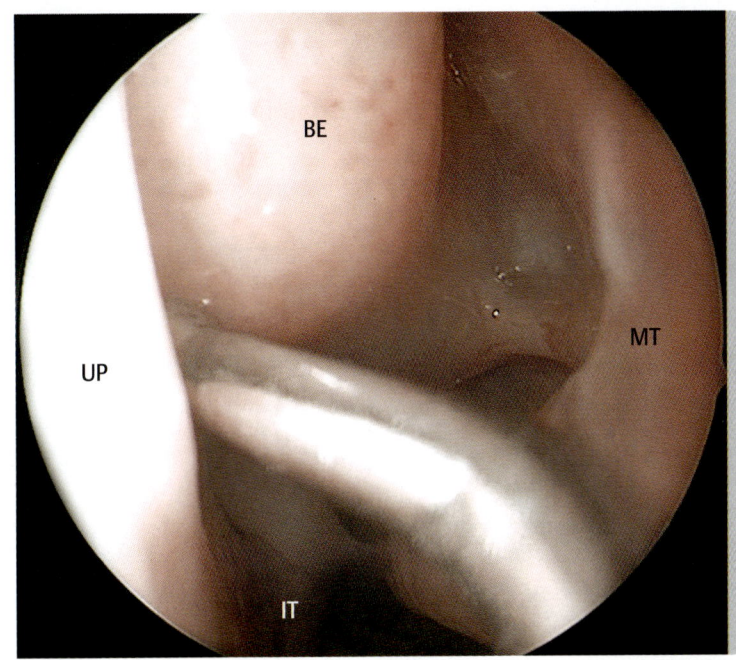

Endoscopic Dissection of the Paranasal Sinuses 43

Fig. 4.3 Ball probe directed into hiatus semilunaris inferioris. BE, bulla ethmoidalis; IT, inferior turbinate; MT, middle turbinate; UP, uncinate process.

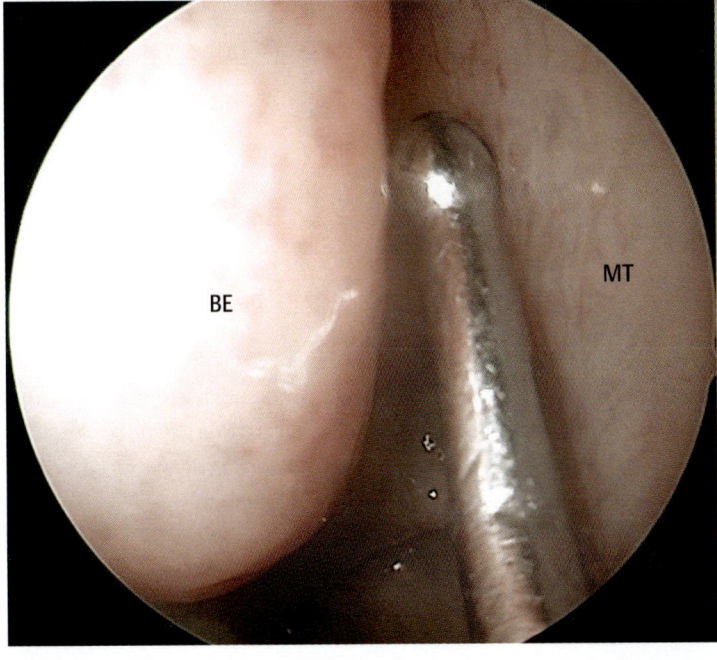

Fig. 4.4 Ball probe directed into hiatus semilunaris superioris. BE, bulla ethmoidalis; MT, middle turbinate.

Technique (Figs. 4.5–4.7)

1. Using a Freer's elevator, the inferior turbinate is lateralized at the level of anterior end of middle turbinate (this increases room for manipulation in middle meatus).
2. Free border of uncinate process is identified.
3. Identification of junction of the upper two-third and lower one-third of the uncinate process which corresponds to the anteroinferior portion of the bulla.
4. With the aid of a backbiting forceps, the uncinate is horizontally cut till the maxillary line.

> **Caution:** Do not bite if resistance/solid bone is encountered.

5. Submucosal dissection of the horizontal portion of the uncinate process is performed.
6. Removal of upper portion of uncinate process is done by passing a probe superiorly along its vertical limb. This helps detach the anterior attachment of the uncinate.
7. Finally, the uncinate is removed till its upper attachment using a microdebrider/90 degrees Blakesley forceps.

> **Caution:**
> - Loss of anatomical architecture of the frontal recess could result from over-zealous plucking/pulling at the upper attachment of the uncinate process. Hence, care must be taken when dissecting the upper part of the uncinate.
> - Additionally, injury to the mucosa in the region of the axilla will eventually lead to scarring and lateralization of middle turbinate.

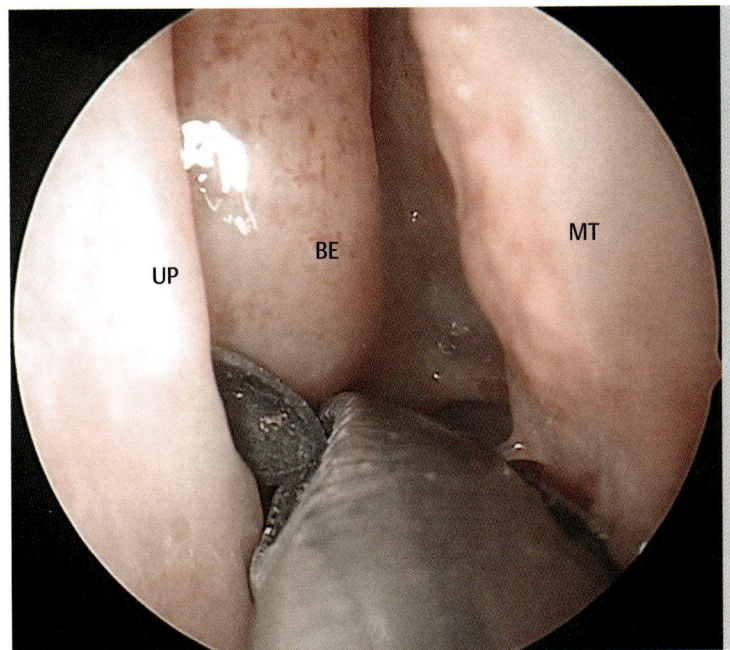

Endoscopic Dissection of the Paranasal Sinuses

Fig. 4.5 Uncinectomy using backbiting forceps. BE, bulla ethmoidalis; MT, middle turbinate; UP, uncinate process.

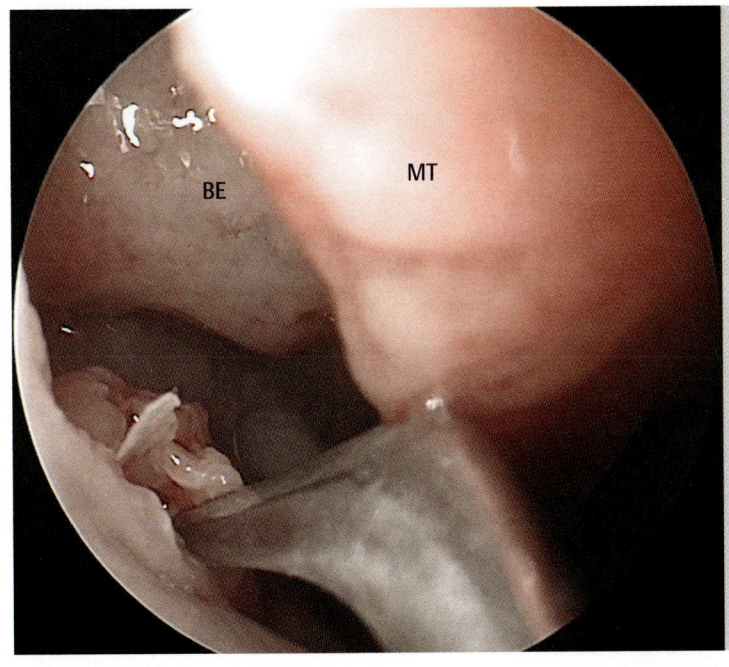

Fig. 4.6 Submucosal dissection of horizontal limb of uncinate. BE, bulla ethmoidalis; MT, middle turbinate.

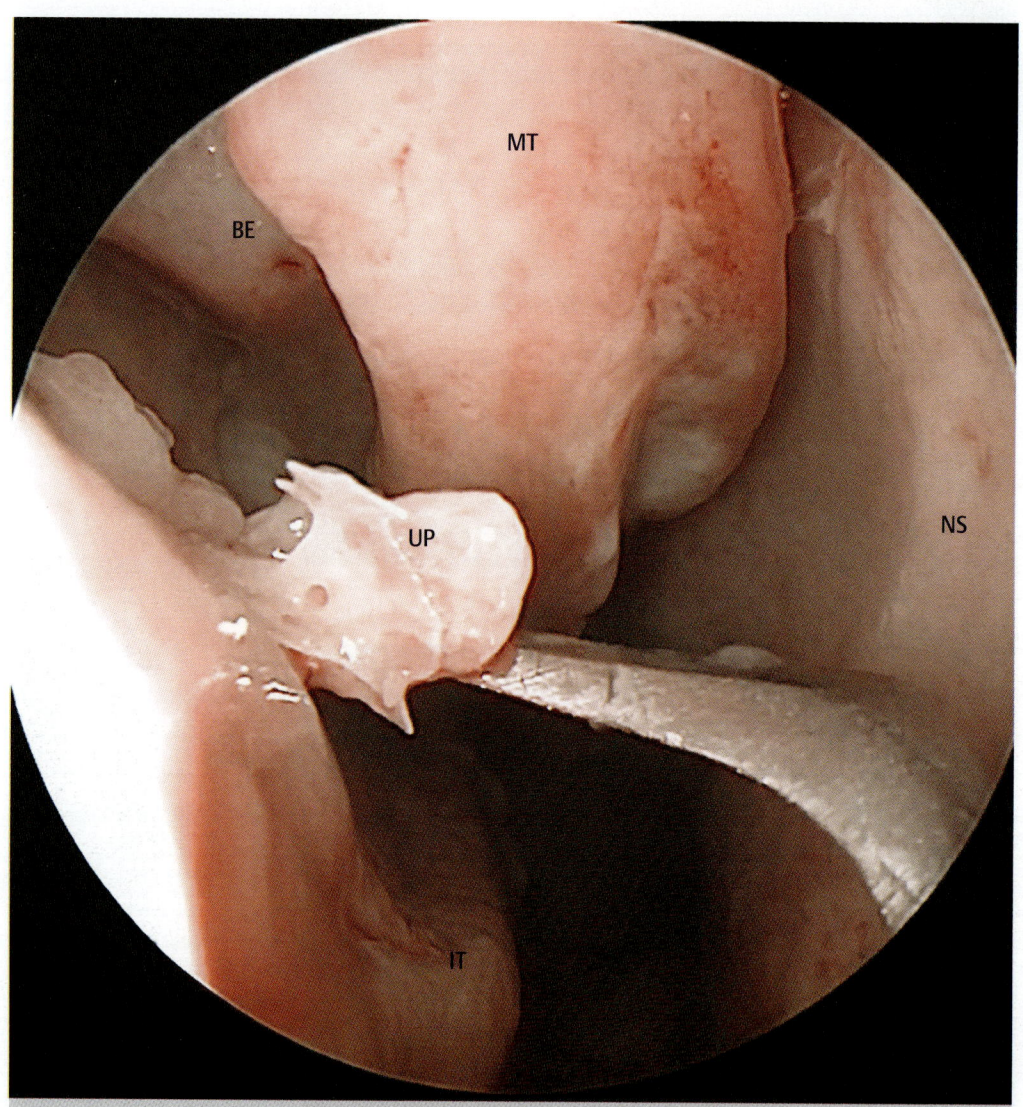

Fig. 4.7 Removal of horizontal limb of uncinate. BE, bulla ethmoidalis; IT, inferior turbinate; MT, middle turbinate; NS, nasal septum; UP, uncinate process.

Middle Meatal Antrostomy (Video 1)

This procedure refers to widening of the natural ostium of maxillary sinus at the cost of the posterior fontanelle.

Technique

A 30- or 45-degree telescope is used to visualize the natural ostium. Conventionally, the ostium is widened using a Blakesley forceps or a microdebrider. This, however, may create raw surfaces circumferentially, resulting in stenosis/closure of the middle meatal antrostomies.[6] This is overcome by the "Uncinate Flap" technique (**Fig. 4.8**).

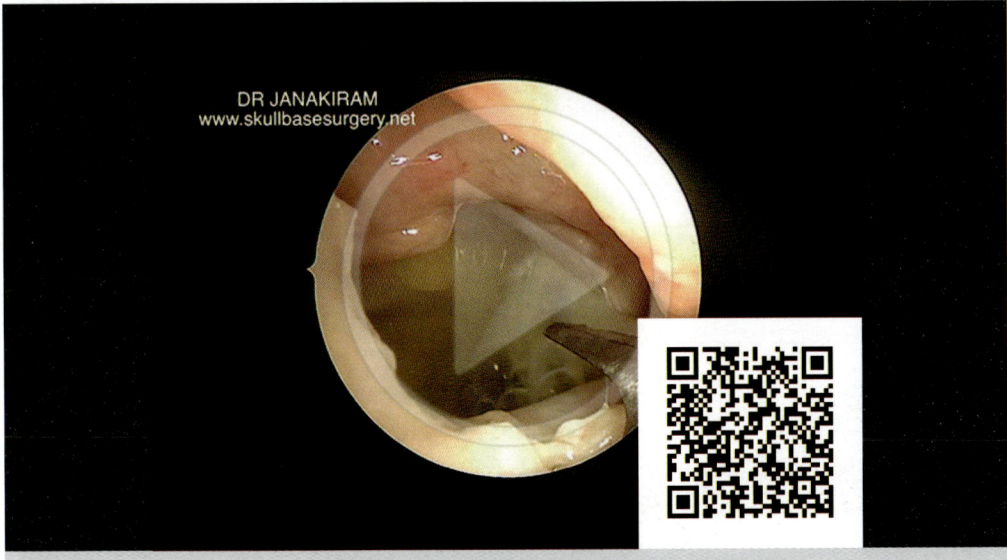

Video 1 Middle meatal antrostomy. https://www.thieme.de/de/q.htm?p=opn/tp/388257077/9789388257060_c001_v001&t=video

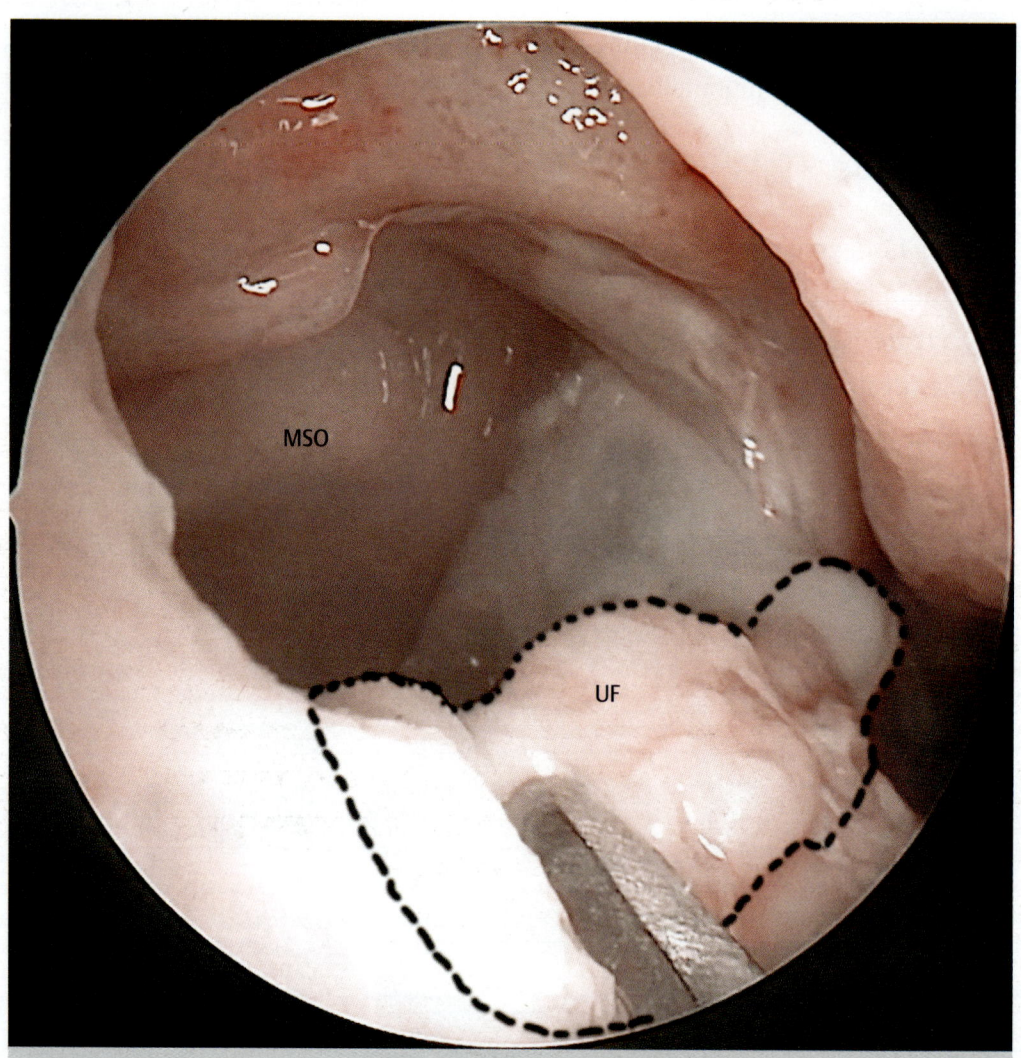

Fig. 4.8 Uncinate flap. UF, uncinate flap; MSO, maxillary sinus ostium.

Endoscopic Dissection of the Paranasal Sinuses

The mucosa on the medial surface of the horizontal portion of the uncinate is debrided. Following this, the horizontal portion of uncinate bone is dissected away with a sickle knife and mucosa of the lateral surface of uncinate is retained.

A scissor is used to cut the mucosa posteriorly and flush with the roof of the maxillary sinus as far back as the accessory ostium and another vertical cut is made at the anterior end of the horizontal limb of the uncinate.

An inferiorly based uncinate flap is created which can be draped over the raw surface created over the superior aspect of the inferior turbinate. The author has observed stenosis rates of < 5% with the use of this flap.

Using a 45-degree telescope, the interior of the maxillary sinus can be examined completely (**Fig. 4.9**).

Some practical guidelines are followed at the author's center for making a middle meatal antrostomy. The horizontal uncinate bone attached to superior border of the inferior turbinate is excised and this defines the lower limit of the antrostomy. Similarly, superiorly the limit is the junction of the orbital lamina of the ethmoid (i.e., lamina papyracea) and the roof of the maxillary sinus. The antrostomy can be extended posteriorly till the posterior wall of the maxillary sinus without damaging any vital structures. Anteriorly, the vertical uncinate is removed with a probe and the mucosal over the uncinate is taken with minimal damage to the mucosal over the hard bone of the nasolacrimal duct. The maxillary ostium is connected to the accessory ostium, if such condition is encountered during the dissection.

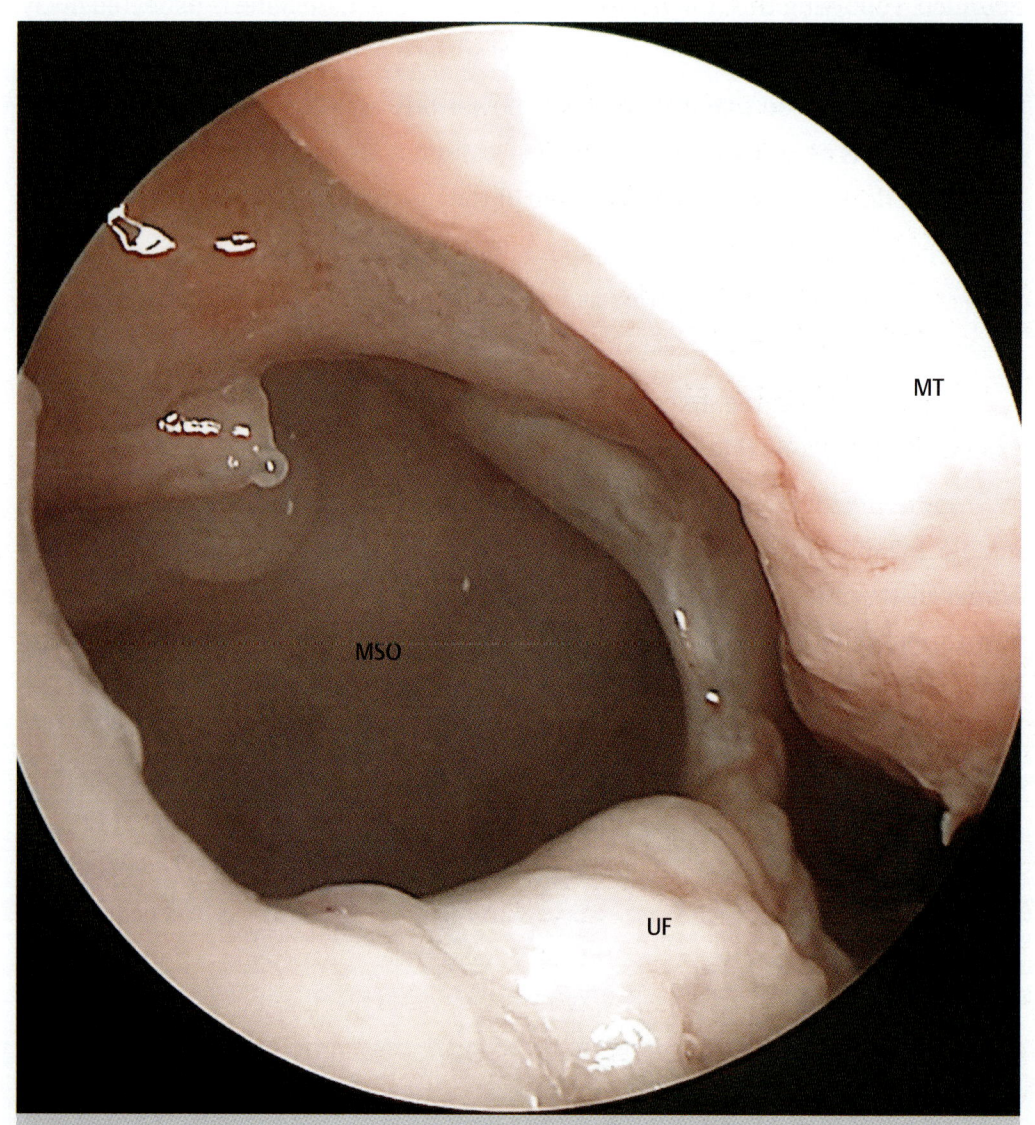

Fig. 4.9 Middle meatal antrostomy. UF, uncinate flap; MSO, maxillary sinus ostium; MT, middle turbinate.

The Frontal Sinus Recess

The frontal recess forms the ethmoidal prechamber to the frontal sinus. FESS primarily involves clearance of frontal recess. The noninflammatory pathologies like tumors of the frontal sinus generally require a larger exposure which is achieved by Draf procedures. The anterior ethmoidal fovea and the frontal recess are regions of extreme anatomical variability. This is because the boundaries of frontal recess are formed by adjunction of four separate anatomical structures:

- The lamina papyracea
- The junction of the middle turbinate and lateral lamina of the cribriform plate
- The frontal beak with agger nasi
- The anterior ethmoidal artery

Similarly, the pneumatization of the frontal bone with the ethmoidal air cells and their relationship with the frontal recess and the orbit give rise to unique anatomical formations described in the following text.

Agger Nasi Cell

This is the anterior most ethmoidal cell formed by pneumatization of the frontal beak. This forms the anterior boundary of the frontal recess, and the agger nasi expands at the expense of the frontal recess; however, it is noteworthy that a big agger will result in a wide frontal recess after removal during surgery (as compared with a smaller agger and a thicker, less pneumatized frontal beak).

Supra-agger/Frontal/Frontoethmoidal Cells

These are single or a tier of cells that are present in the frontal recess and can extend up to the frontal sinus. They can also completely lie in the frontal sinus. Kuhn classified these cells in to four types:

- **Type 1:** Single frontal recess cell above agger nasi cell
- **Type 2:** Tier of cells in frontal recess above agger nasi cell
- **Type 3:** Single massive cell pneumatizing cephalad into frontal sinus
- **Type 4 (modified from original classification):** A cell pneumatizing through into the frontal sinus and extending > 50% of the vertical height of the frontal sinus

Suprabullar Cell

A cell present above the bulla, not extending into the frontal sinus, with its posterior wall formed by skull base.

Supraorbital Ethmoidal Cell

An anterior ethmoidal cell that pneumatizes over the orbit making the anterior ethmoidal artery dehisent is a supraorbital ethmoidal cell.[7]

Frontal Recess Dissection (Video 2)

The boundaries of the frontal recess are:
- **Anteriorly:** Agger nasi
- **Posteriorly:** Anterior ethmoidal artery
- **Medially:** Middle turbinate
- **Laterally:** Lamina papyracea

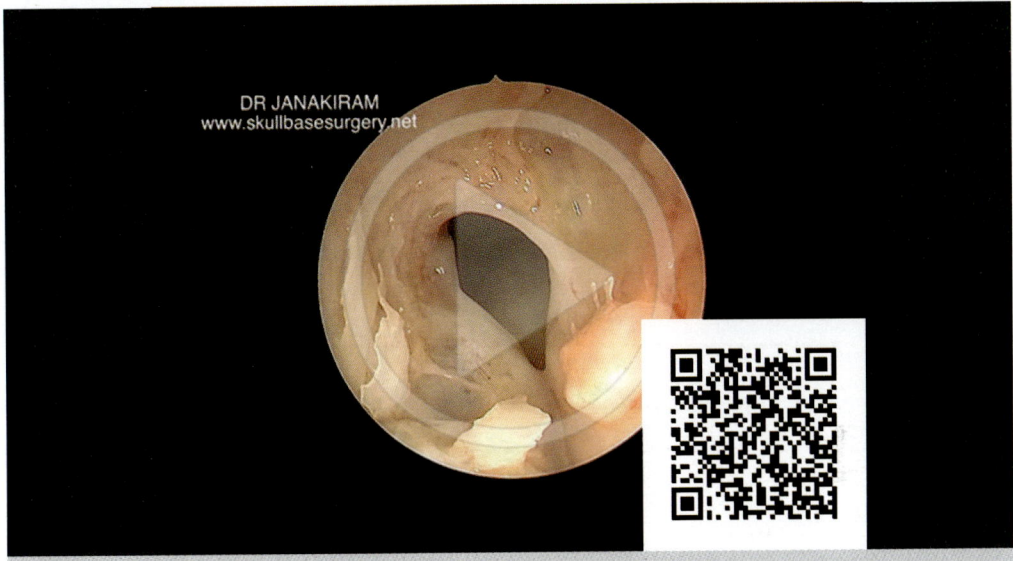

Video 2 Frontal recess dissection. https://www.thieme.de/de/q.htm?p=opn/tp/388257077/9789388257060_c001_v002&t=video

Technique[8] (Figs. 4.10–4.13)

This section describes the intact bulla technique wherein the frontal recess is opened before opening of the bulla. Injury to the anterior ethmoidal artery is unlikely with this technique as the upper attachment of the bulla lies anterior to the vessel. Using a 45-degree telescope, the agger nasi cell is located. A frontal ball probe is then slid between the upper attachment of middle turbinate and the agger nasi (posterior and medial to agger nasi cell).

Agger nasi is gently pushed forward and laterally with utmost care and respect to the mucosa. This opens up the frontal sinus. Transillumination of frontal sinus can now be appreciated. The frontal drainage pathway described here is called medial drainage and is seen in 70% of individuals.

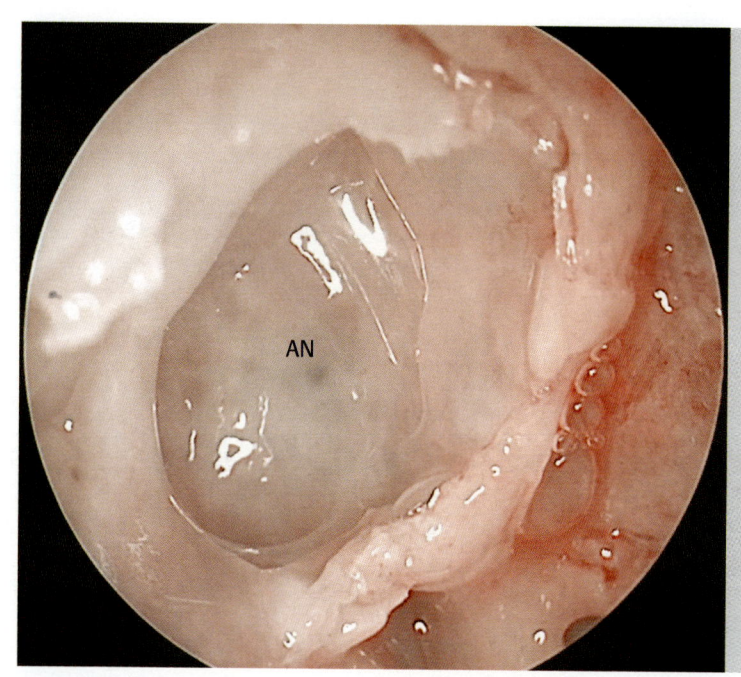

Fig. 4.10 Agger nasi seen after removal of vertical limb of uncinate. AN, agger nasi.

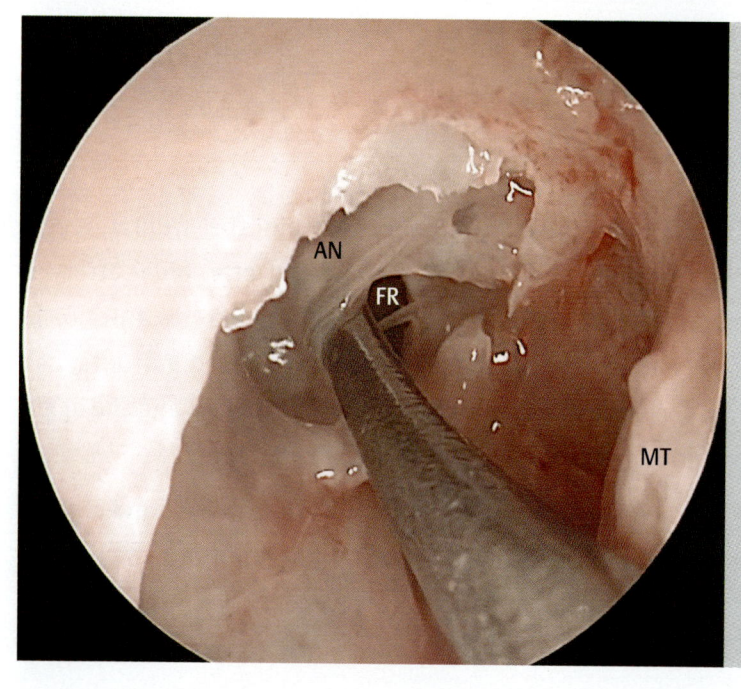

Fig. 4.11 Uncapping of agger nasi to visualize frontal recess. AN, agger nasi; FR, frontal recess; MT, middle turbinate.

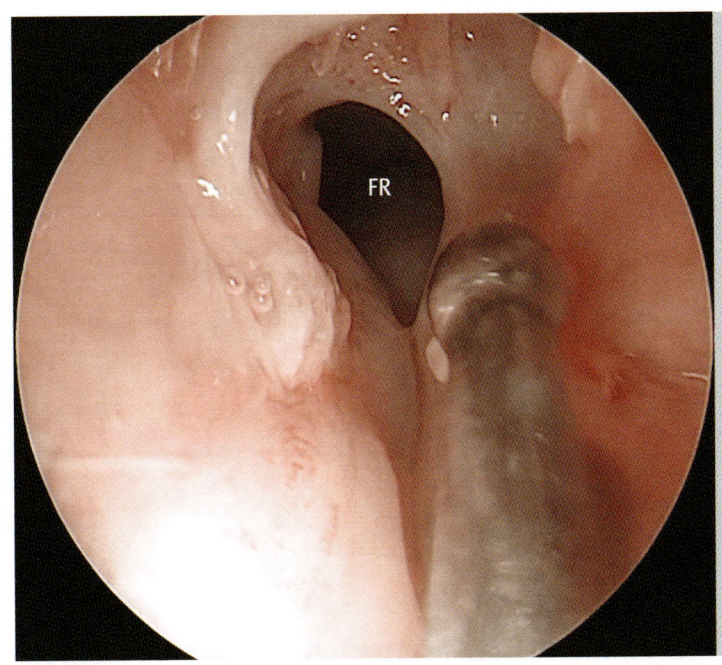

Endoscopic Dissection of the Paranasal Sinuses

Fig. 4.12 Frontal recess seen after removal of anterior and medial wall of agger nasi. FR, frontal recess.

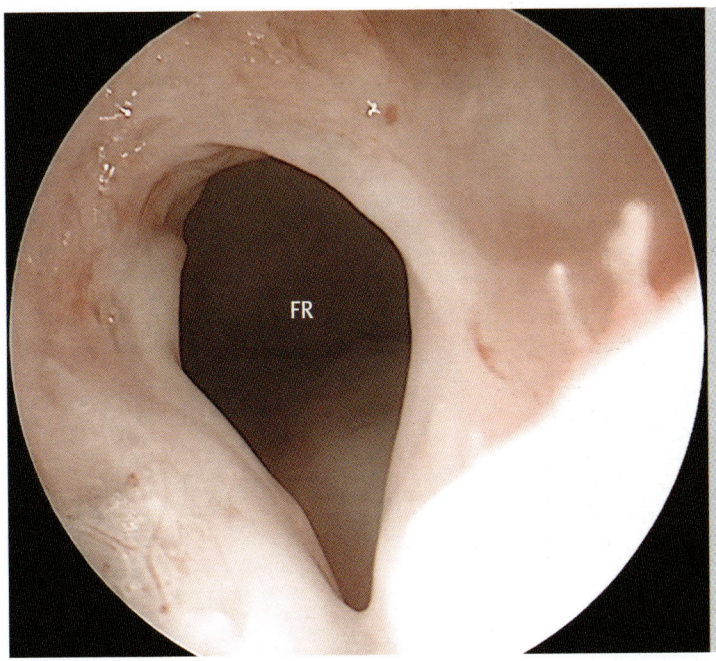

Fig. 4.13 Frontal sinus visualized through frontal recess. FR, frontal recess.

In other cases, the frontal recess is approached tracing the fovea from posterior to anterior from the sphenoid osteum. The frontal recess is generally located anterior to the anterior fovea. The frontal recess lies immediate anterior to or a cell anterior to the anterior ethmoidal canal.

Note: The frontal drainage pathway in an individual is determined by the attachment of the uncinate. If the uncinate gets attached to the middle turbinate/skull base, the frontal sinus drains directly into the infundibulum. This is described as lateral drainage.

Dissection of Anterior Ethmoid (Video 3)

The bulla is the largest anterior ethmoid cell. It consists of six walls:

- Anterior wall
- Medial wall (related to the lateral wall of hiatus semilunaris superioris)

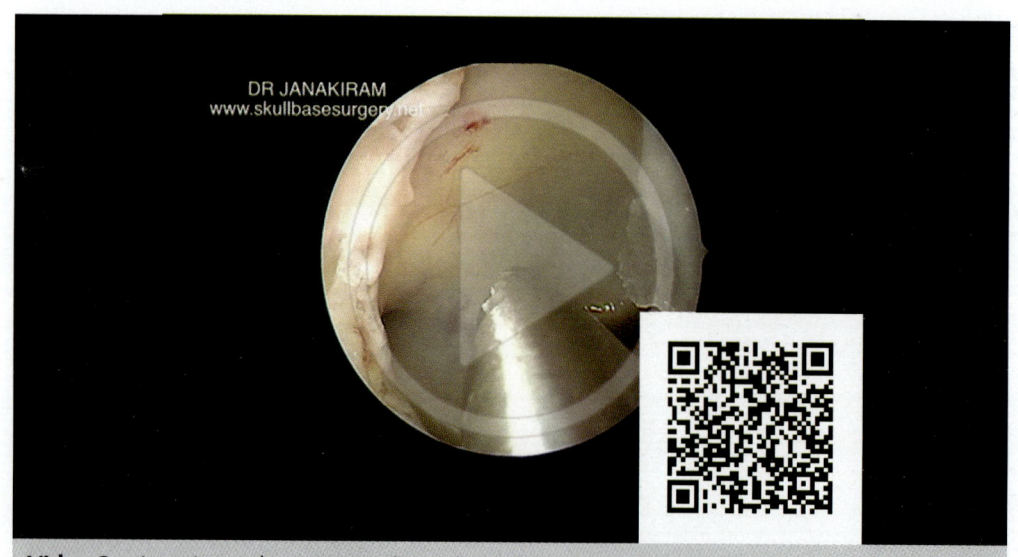

Video 3 Anterior and posterior ethmoidectomy, sphenoidotomy, and skull base dissection. https://www.thieme.de/de/q.htm?p=opn/tp/388257077/9789388257060_c001_v003&t=video

- Lateral wall (lamina papyracea)
- Posterior wall (related to retrobullar recess)
- Superior wall (could be attached to skull base/related to suprabullar recess)
- Inferior wall

Technique

1. Following identification of the anterior wall of the bulla, it is opened anteroinferiorly using a microdebrider/Blakesley forceps (**Fig. 4.14**).
2. With the aid of a 45-degree telescope, the skull base is examined. Inability to visualize the skull base after opening the bulla indicates the presence of suprabullar cells. These cells may be carefully removed using a microdebrider/frontal ball probe.
3. After clearing all anterior ethmoidal cells, the following structures are seen:
    a. Anterior ethmoidal neurovascular bundle running obliquely from posterior to anterior, and lateral to medial direction.
    b. Small portion of anterior fovea between posterior wall of frontal sinus and anterior ethmoidal artery.

It is vital to understand that during the dissection of anterior ethmoidal cells, the presence of suprabullar or a supraorbital cell increases the chances of a dehiscent anterior ethmoidal canal and an inadvertent injury to the anterior ethmoidal artery while clearing the roof. Another important aspect is that while addressing the lateral wall of the bulla, clearance of this wall should be done in a direction parallel to (i.e., anteroposterior) to the lamina papyracea.

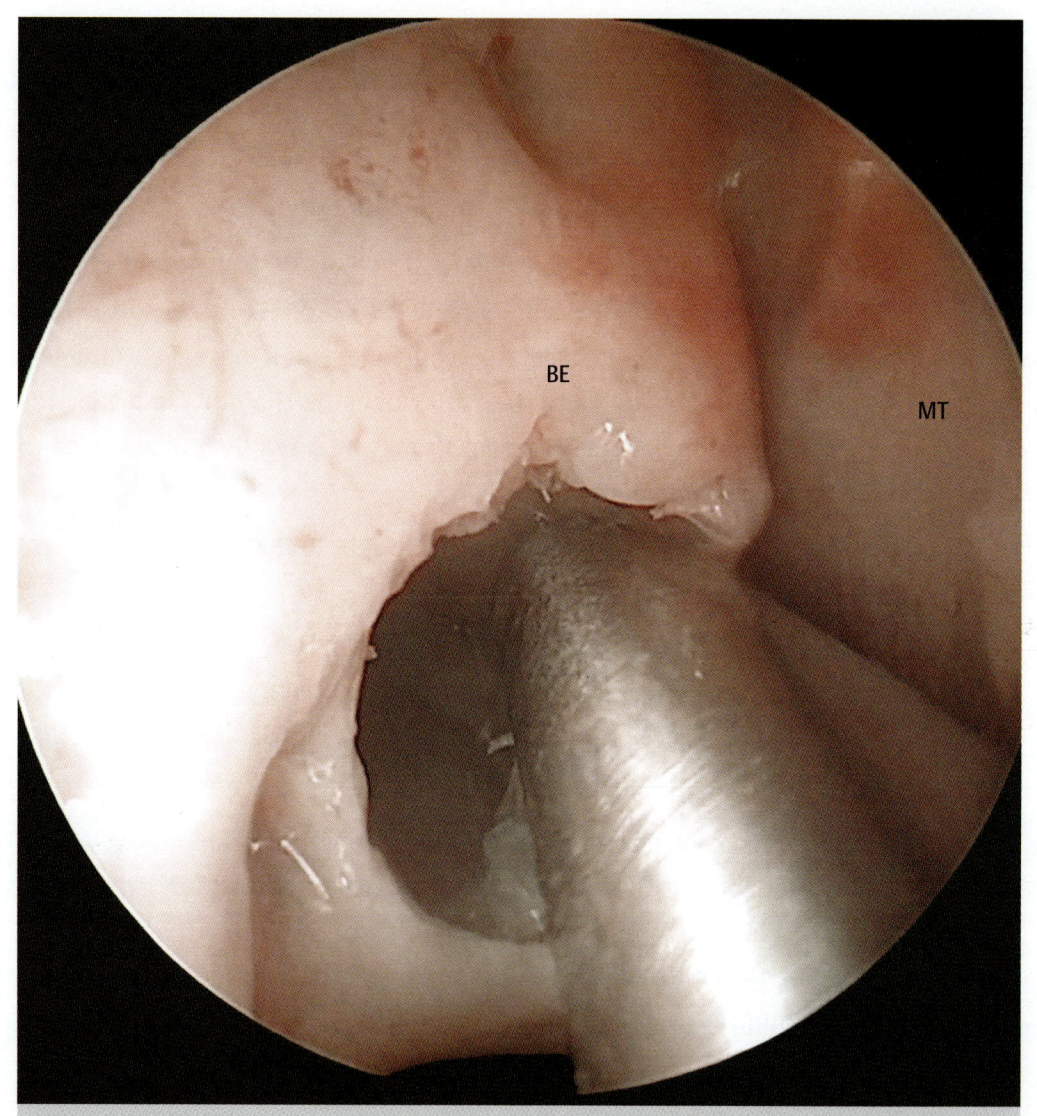

Fig. 4.14 The bulla is opened inferomedially. BE, bulla ethmoidalis; MT, middle turbinate.

Dissection of Posterior Ethmoid (Video 3)

Boundaries of the posterior ethmoid include:

- Anteriorly: Ground lamella
- Posteriorly: Anterior wall of sphenoid sinus
- Laterally: Lamina papyracea
- Superiorly: Posterior skull base
- Medially: Superior turbinate

Technique

1. A Blakesley forceps is gently slide along the horizontal attachment of middle turbinate after identification ground lamella.
2. The basal lamella is perforated medially and inferiorly using the forceps (**Fig. 4.15**).
3. All cells are removed till the posterior skull base is identified.

> **Note:** The skull base descends inferiorly toward in its posterior aspect. The lamina papyracea is yellowish in appearance in comparison to the pearly white color of the skull base where the posterior ethmoidal neurovascular bundle is seen.

Like the anterior ethmoids, dissection in this region along the lateral wall is focused to delineate the lamina and the optic nerve in its posterior part. The variation in the posterior most of the posterior ethmoid cells that pneumatized in to the sphenoid sinus is called as sphenoethmoid or an Onodi cell. Such a cell may have the optic nerve canal on its lateral aspect. Such is cell is better detected on a preoperative computed tomography.

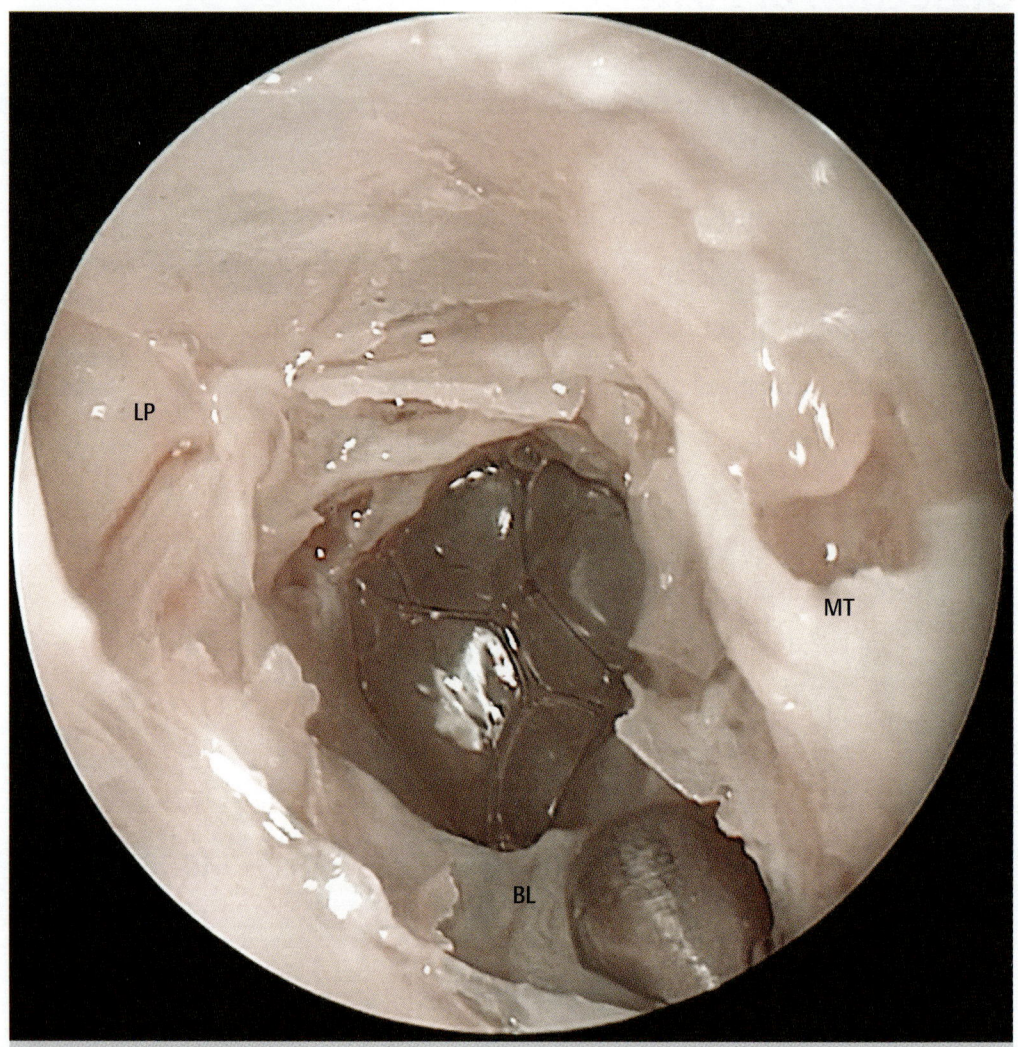

Fig. 4.15 Opening basal lamella to enter posterior ethmoidal cells. BL, basal lamella; LP, lamina papyracea; MT, middle turbinate.

Dissection of Sphenoid Sinus (Video 3)

There are three routes to approach the sphenoid sinus:
1. Lateral approach: Dissecting posterior–inferior and medial to the posterior ethmoid.
2. Intermediate approach: Creating a superior meatal window.
3. Medial approach: Lateralizing the middle turbinate and approaching the sphenoid os.

Intermediate Approach

1. The inferior wall of bulla is followed backward toward posterior end of middle turbinate.
2. A microdebrider is then used directing the blade medially taking care not to damage the septal mucosa.
3. The anterior end of superior turbinate is identified and is gently pushed laterally to identify the sphenoid os (**Fig. 4.16**).
4. A Silcut forceps is used to resect the inferior third of superior turbinate (**Fig. 4.17**).
5. The sphenoid os is now visualized and is widened using Stammberger mushroom punch.

The following structures are identified in the sphenoid sinus (**Fig. 4.18**):
- Orbital apex
- Optic nerve
- Internal carotid artery
- Sellar floor

Note the position of the posterior ethmoidal artery in relation to the anterior wall of the sphenoid sinus.

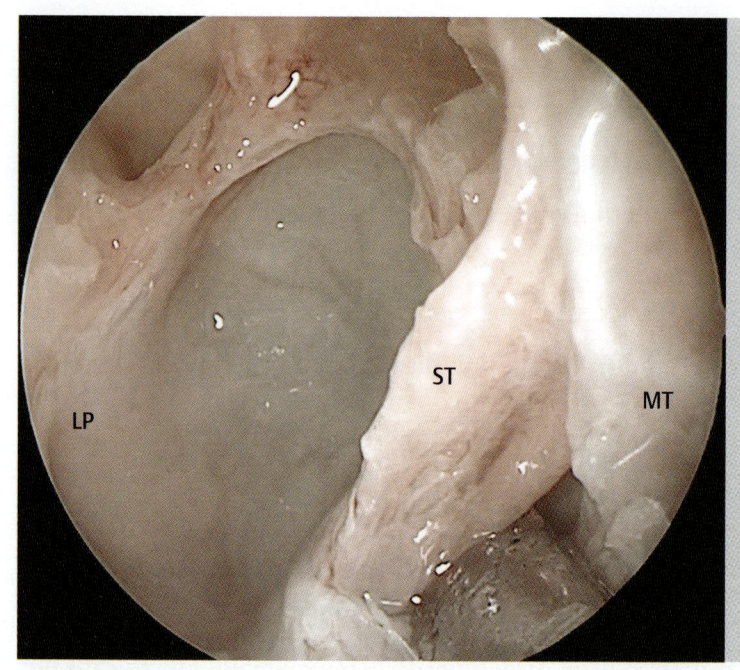

Fig. 4.16 Superior meatal window. LP, lamina papyracea; MT, middle turbinate; ST, superior turbinate.

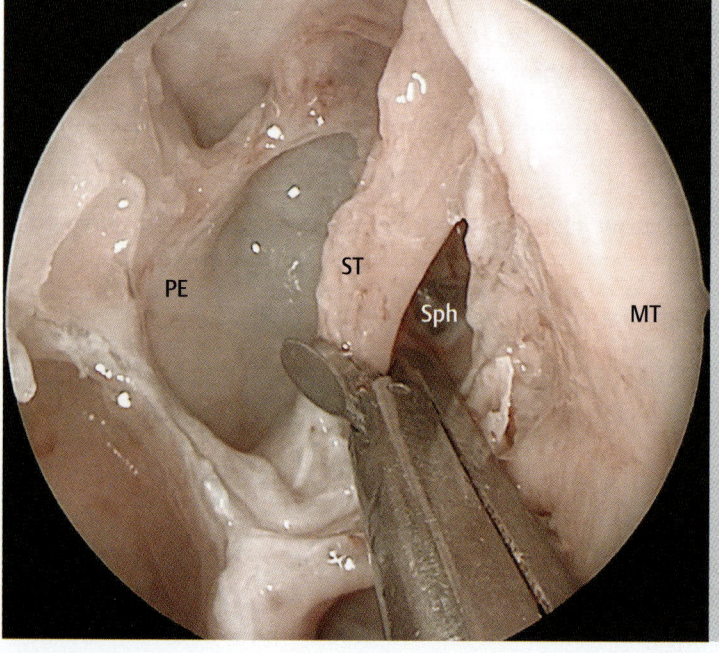

Fig. 4.17 Truncate lower one-third of superior turbinate. MT, middle turbinate; PE, posterior ethmoid; Sph, sphenoid sinus; ST, superior turbinate.

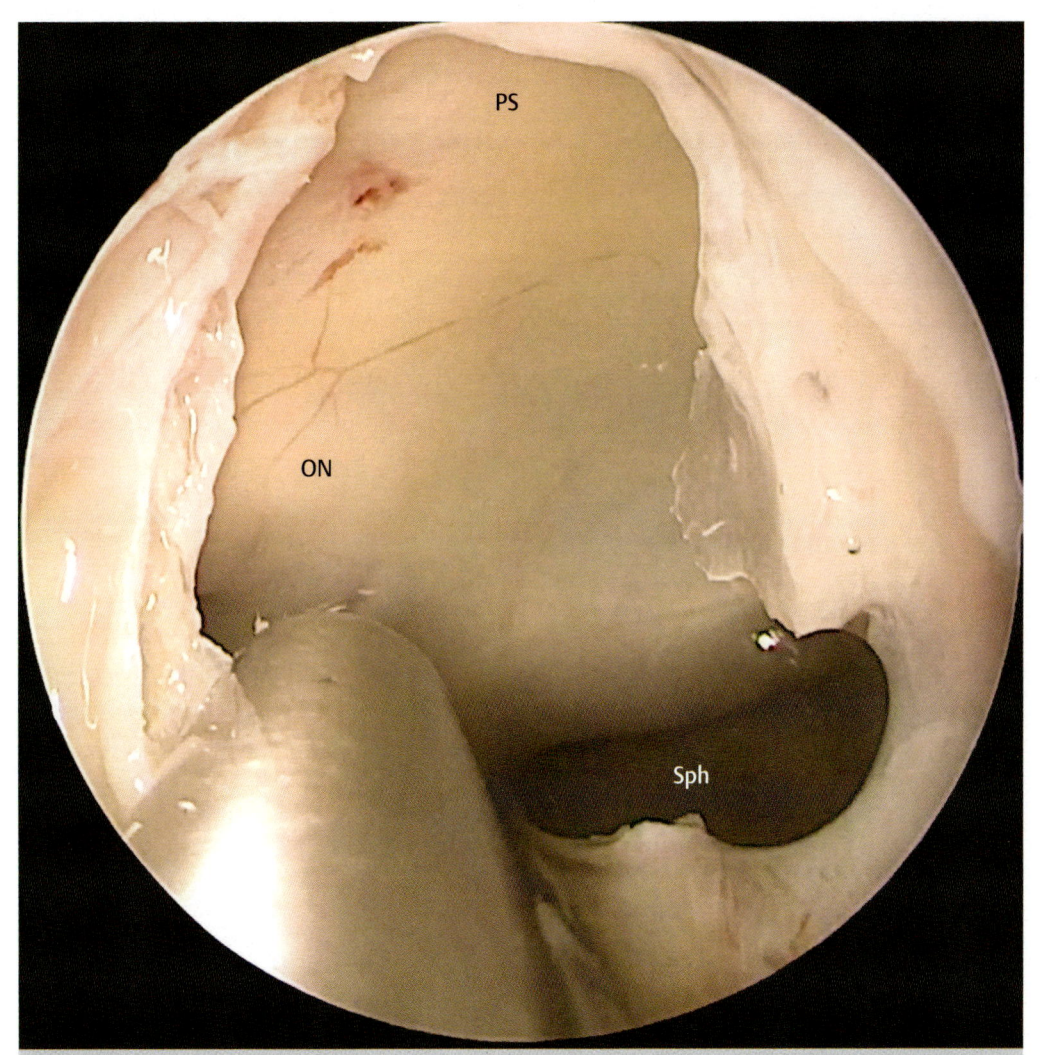

Endoscopic Dissection of the Paranasal Sinuses

Fig. 4.18 Widening sphenoid sinus. ON, optic nerve; PS, planum sphenoidale; Sph, sphenoid sinus.

Once the complete dissection is done, identification of various structures of skull base from posterior to anterior is done (**Figs. 4.19–4.20**):

- Posterior ethmoidal neurovascular bundle
    - Posterior fovea

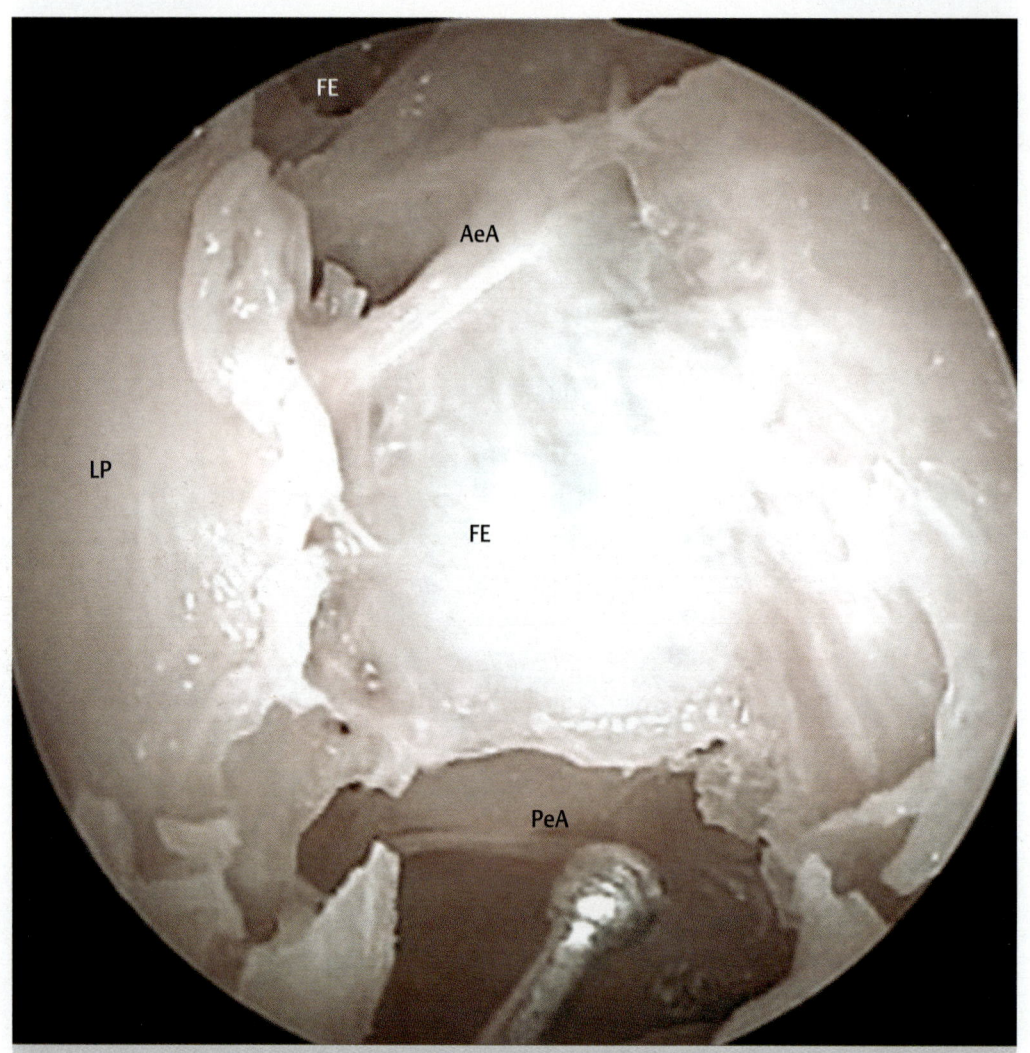

Fig. 4.19 Skull base. AeA, anterior ethmoidal artery; FE, fovea ethmoidalis; LP, lamina papyracea; PeA, posterior ethmoidal artery.

Endoscopic Dissection of the Paranasal Sinuses

- Anterior ethmoidal neurovascular bundle
  - Anterior fovea
  - Frontal recess

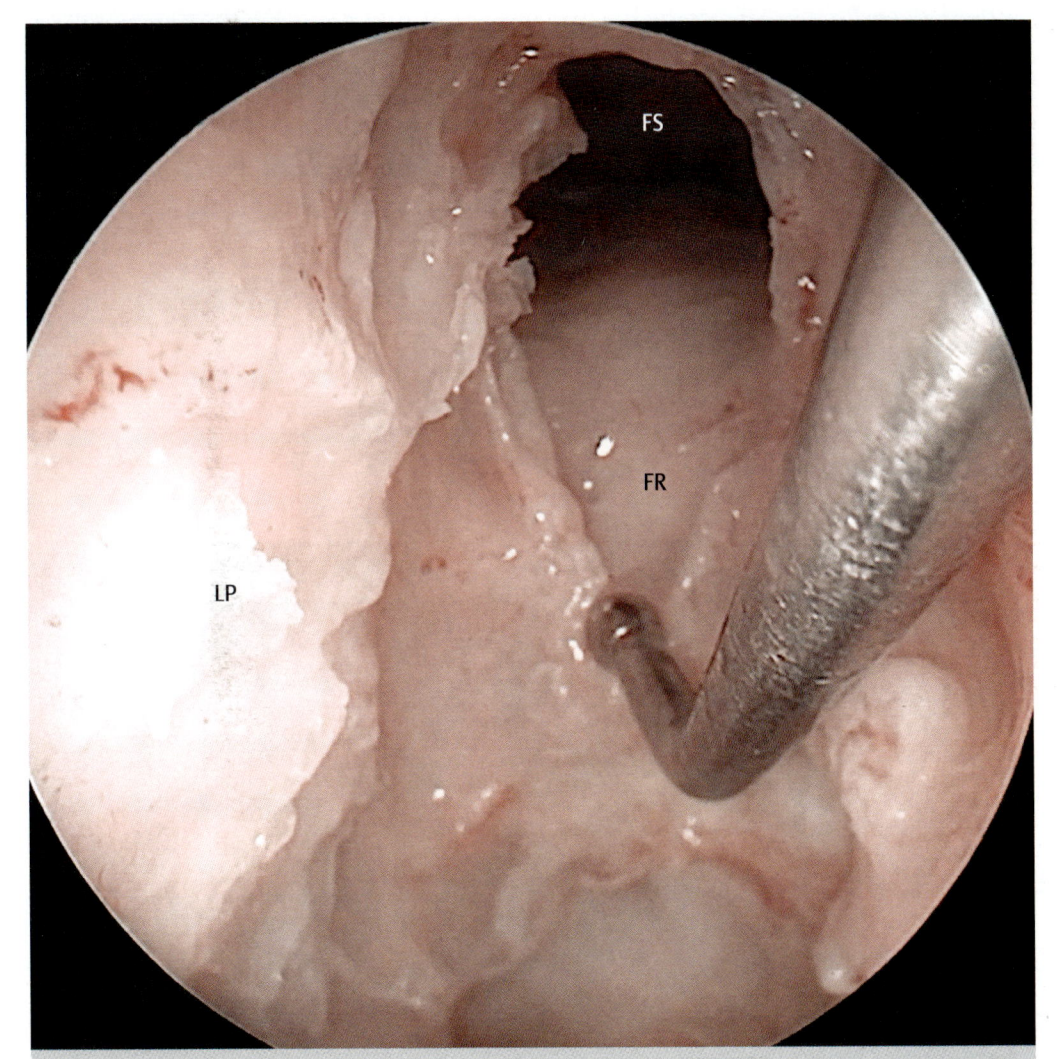

Fig. 4.20 Widened frontal recess. FR, frontal recess; FS, frontal sinus; LP, lamina papyracea.

Endoscopic Dacryocystorhinostomy—Modified Approach (Video 4)

The lacrimal sac is located in the lateral nasal wall anterior to middle turbinate with its upper margin extends above the attachment of middle turbinate. The maxillary line helps identify the lacrimal sac and appears as a prominence between the axilla of the middle meatus and the inferior turbinate. The use of an inferiorly based mucosal flap is different from the technique described by Wormold.[9] Placement of the mucosal flap inferiorly is crucial to the success of this technique, as it ensures full exposure of the sac.[9] The flap promotes early mucosalisation, without hindering the procedure. During this procedure, no bone is left exposed and granulations are minimal; hence, excellent healing by primary intention is observed.

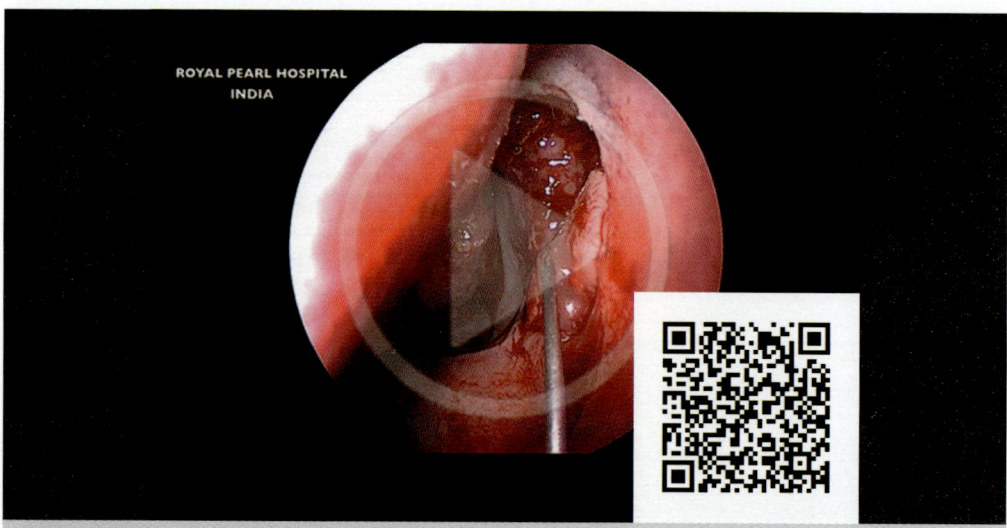

Video 4 Endoscopic DCR—our technique. https://www.thieme.de/de/q.htm?p=opn/tp/388257077/9789388257060_c001_v004&t=video

Endoscopic Dissection of the Paranasal Sinuses

Technique[10]

1. A 0-degree 4-mm endoscope is used for the procedure.
2. An inferiorly based flap is raised in the lateral nasal wall to expose the lacrimal bone and the frontal process of the maxilla using a knife.
3. A superior incision is placed just above the axilla of the middle turbinate and an anterior incision is placed 8 mm anterior to the axilla of the middle turbinate, which is in front of the uncinate, posteriorly (**Fig. 4.21**).
4. A 0.5 × 0.5 cm section of the mucosa in the flap in front of axilla is incised and removed using a Rosen elevator or a blade. This is the mucosa overlying the lacrimal sac. The Rosen elevator is used to gently elevate the flap from the bone in an anterior to posterior direction. From the posterior edge, the flap is gently pulled in the inferior direction to free it from nasal mucosa using Blakesley forceps. The use of suction is avoided.

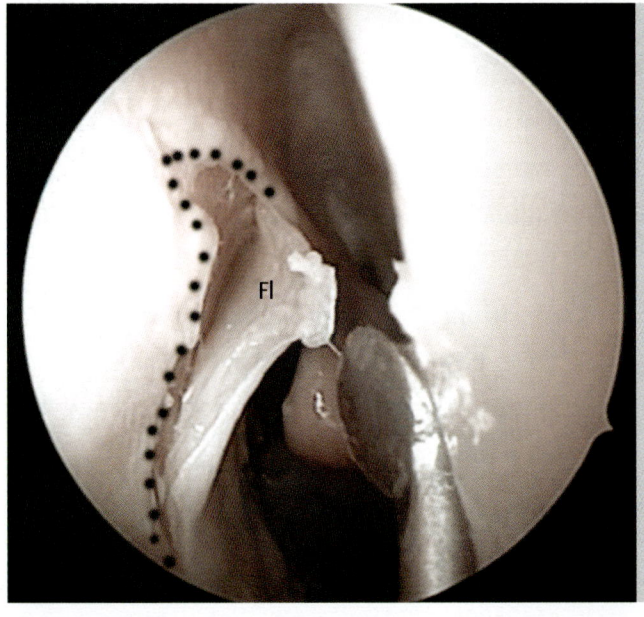

Fig. 4.21 Incision marking for flap. Fl, flap.

5. The inferiorly based flap is rotated on itself and placed on the inferior turbinate (**Fig. 4.22**). Any adhesions to the bone or nasal mucosa are cut using scissors.

6. The frontal process of the maxilla is nibbled in a posterior to anterior direction, just above the flap, to the anterior edge, using a 2 mm Kerrison rongeur (**Fig. 4.23**). Traction is maintained medially to prevent pressure injury to the lacrimal sac during this process.

7. Drilling is conducted using a DCR burr to remove the superior thick bone and expose the fundus of the sac, without applying pressure, thereby avoiding lacrimal sac injury. The thin lacrimal bone is gently elevated from the lacrimal sac. Complete bone removal is ensured (**Fig. 4.24**).

8. After removal of bone, the endosteal layer is observed on the medial wall of the sac (**Fig. 4.24**).

9. In the modified technique, removal of the endosteal layer is performed separately from that of the endothelial layer of the sac. The endosteal layer is removed with a sickle knife, gently and in a downward direction (**Fig. 4.25**).

10. The medial wall is then incised using a number 11 blade, allowing the accumulated pus to drain. Anterior and posterior flaps of the medial wall of the sac are created, thus marsupializing the lacrimal sac. Canalicular openings are visualized. Syringing is performed to remove mucus plugs and ensure patency.

11. The inferiorly based flap is repositioned and approximated with the nasal mucosa so that no bone is left exposed (**Fig. 4.26**). The anteriorly based lacrimal sac flap is repositioned on the inferiorly based flap and the posterior sac flap is placed on the uncinate.

Note: Lasers, radio frequency ablation, removal of mucosal flap, and diathermy are not recommended as all these have high failure rates.

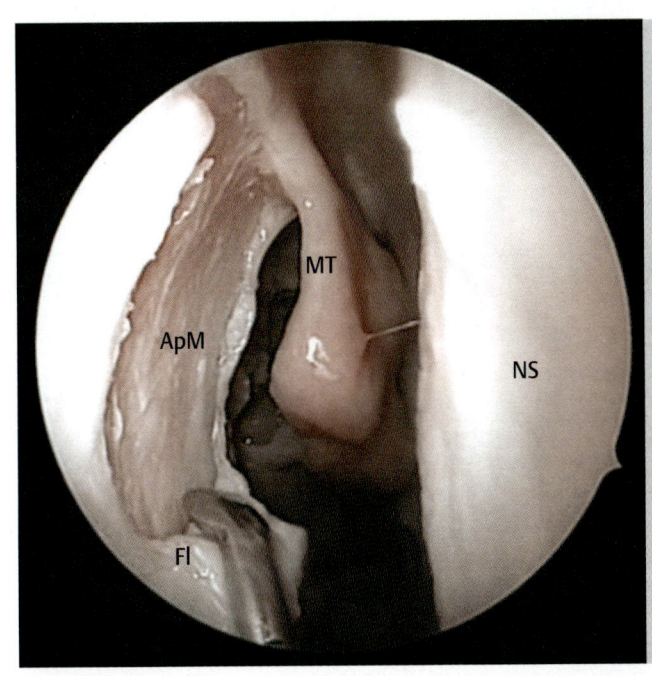

Endoscopic Dissection of the Paranasal Sinuses 69

Fig. 4.22 Inferiorly based mucosal flap. ApM, ascending process of maxilla; Fl, flap; MT, middle turbinate; NS, nasal septum.

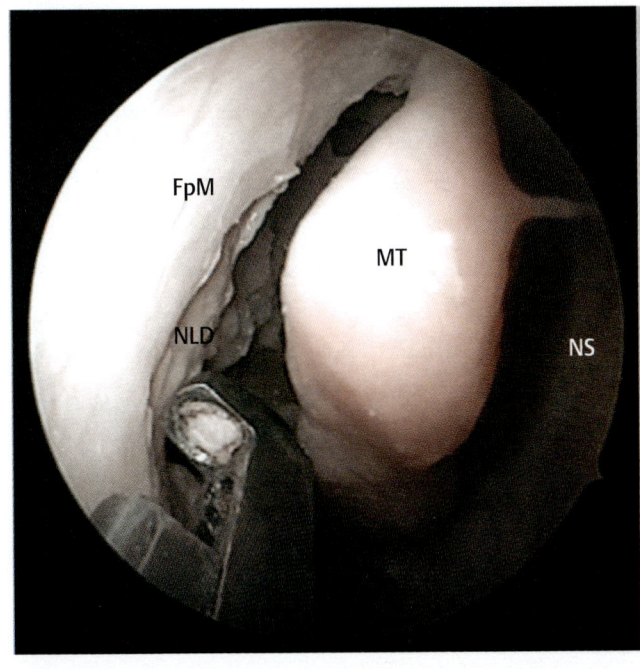

Fig. 4.23 Frontal process of maxilla punched out and nasolacrimal duct exposed. FpM, frontal process of maxilla; MT, middle turbinate; NLD, nasolacrimal duct; NS, nasal septum.

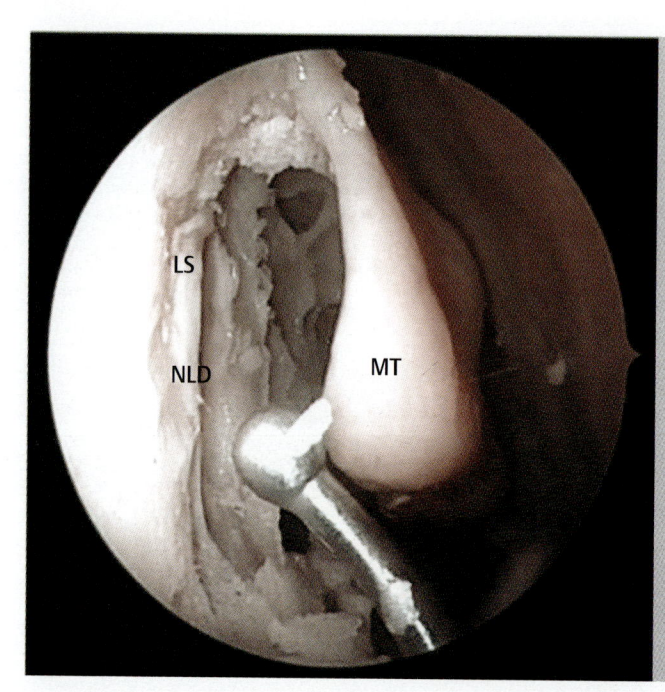

Fig. 4.24 Lacrimal sac and nasolacrimal duct exposed. LS, lacrimal sac; MT, middle turbinate; NLD, nasolacrimal duct.

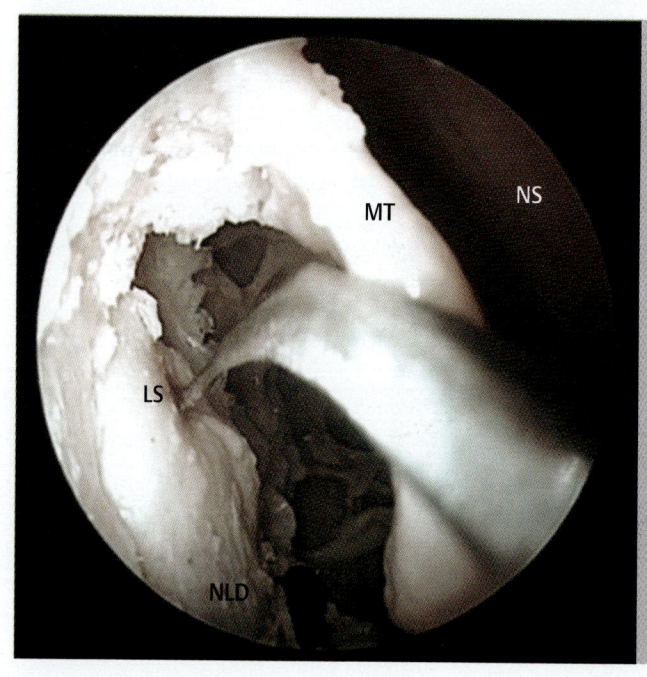

Fig. 4.25 Endosteal layer of lacrimal sac incised. LS, lacrimal sac; MT, middle turbinate; NLD, nasolacrimal duct; NS, nasal septum.

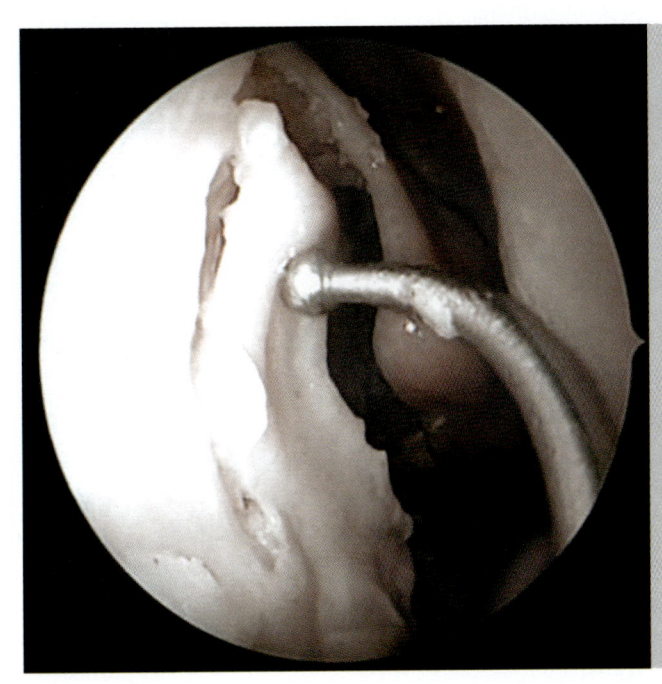

Fig. 4.26 Mucosal flap repositioned.

References

1. Stammberger H, Posawetz W. Functional endoscopic sinus surgery. Concept, indications and results of the Messerklinger technique. Eur Arch Otorhinolaryngol 1990;247(2): 63–76

2. Wormald PJ. The agger nasi cell: the key to understanding the anatomy of the frontal recess. Otolaryngol Head Neck Surg 2003;129(5):497–507

3. Zhang L, Han D, Ge W, et al. Anatomical and computed tomographic analysis of the interaction between the uncinate process and the agger nasi cell. Acta Otolaryngol 2006;126(8):845–852

4. Landsberg R, Friedman M. A computer-assisted anatomical study of the nasofrontal region. Laryngoscope 2001;111(12):2125–2130

5. El-Shazly AE, Poirrier AL, Cabay J, Lefebvre PP. Anatomical variations of the lateral nasal wall: the secondary and accessory middle turbinates. Clin Anat 2012;25(3):340–346

6. Wormald PJ, McDonogh M. The 'swing-door' technique for uncinectomy in endoscopic sinus surgery. J Laryngol Otol 1998;112(6):547–551

7. Wormald PJ, Hoseman W, Callejas C, et al. The International Frontal Sinus Anatomy Classification (IFAC) and Classification of the Extent of Endoscopic Frontal Sinus Surgery (EFSS). Int Forum Allergy Rhinol 2016;6(7):677–696

8. Draf W. Endonasal microendoscopic frontal sinus surgery, the Fulda concept. Oper Tech Otolaryngol--Head Neck Surg 1991;2:234–240

9. Wormald PJ. Powered endoscopic dacryocystorhinostomy. Laryngoscope 2002; 112(1): 69–72

10. Janakiram TN, Suri N, Sharma SB. Modified approach to powered endoscopic dacryocystorhinostomy. J Laryngol Otol 2016;130(3):261–264

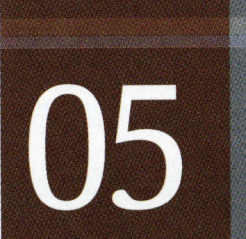

05 Tips and Tricks in Ventral Skull Base Dissection

Narayanan Janakiram, Dharambir S. Sethi, Onkar K. Deshmukh, and Arvindh K. Gananathan

- § Introduction 75
- § General Principles 76

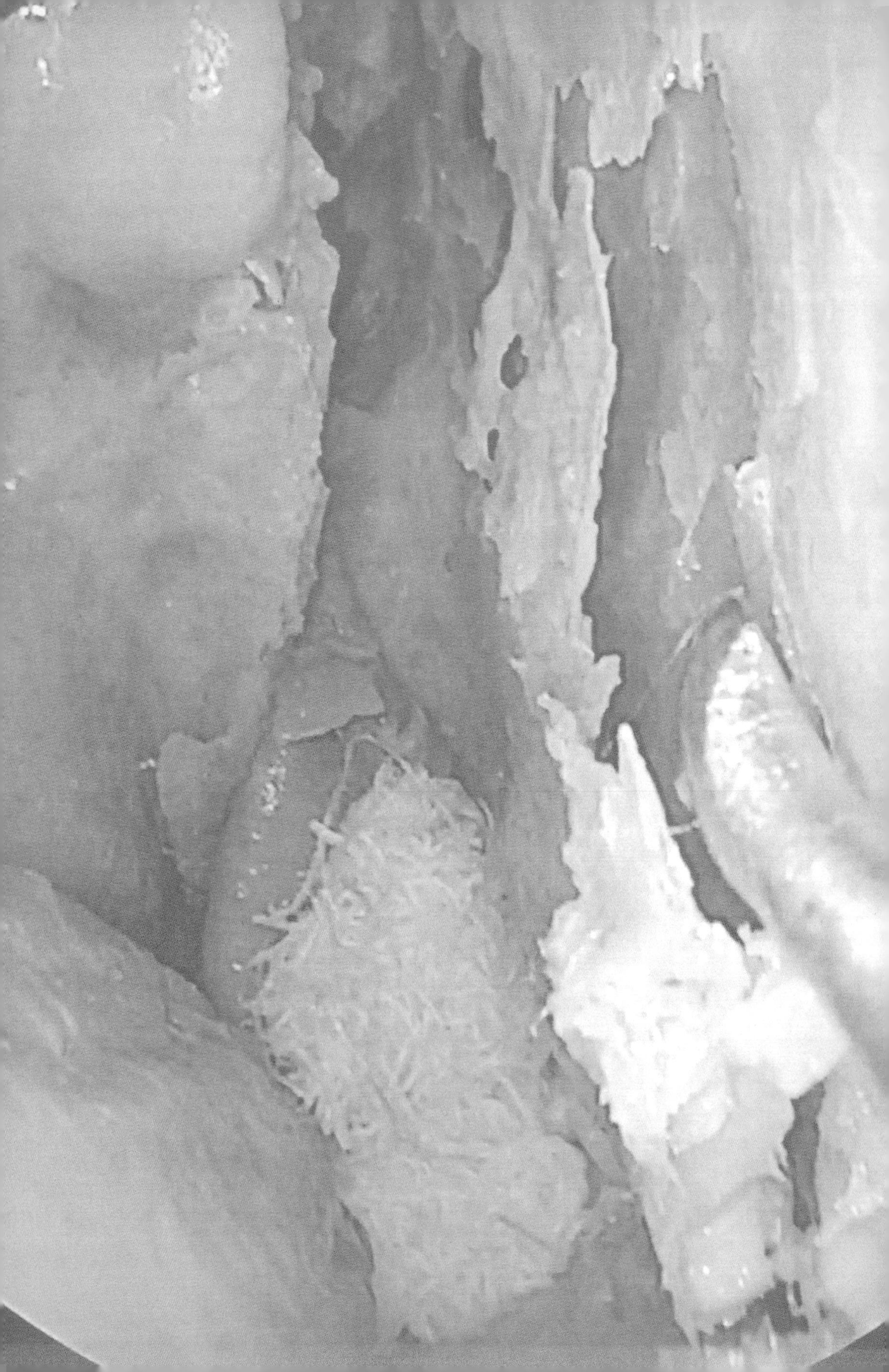

Introduction

Ventral skull base constitutes the complex anatomical watershed between the surgical territories of neurosurgery and otorhinolaryngology. The complexity of anterior skull base anatomy is attributed to its intricate interrelationships with vital neurovascular structures. These are further augmented by the myriad of anatomical variations resulting from the differential pneumatization patterns of the paranasal sinuses.

Endonasal endoscopic approaches provide improved visualization and access to different areas of the ventral skull base, which, in turn, facilitates better tumor clearance. Additional advantages of these approaches are better cosmesis, improved postoperative morbidity, and thus superior surgical outcomes. Accurate orientation to endoscopic anatomy, thorough knowledge of anatomical variations, surgical expertise, and appropriate instrumentation are the primal prerequisites for dealing with skull base pathologies via these approaches.

Mastering sophisticated endoscopic skull base techniques translates into superior surgical outcome. This can be best achieved by continued endoscopic cadaveric skull base dissections. Anatomical dissections enable the dissector to familiarize with the irregular bony topography, two-dimensional views, and also help acquire appropriate practical skills. These orient the trainees/dissectors to identify important anatomical landmarks and avoid critical neurovascular structures.

Another vital aspect in skull base training is in-depth understanding of imaging studies. Computed tomography (CT) scans aid in identifying anatomical variations and also in consolidating a roadmap for skull base surgery. Tumor extension and soft tissue involvement can be better mapped on a magnetic resonance imaging (MRI). Repeated comparison for endoscopic picture with a coronal CT scan helps maintain surgical orientation at all times. It is vital for a skull base surgeon to develop the ability to reconstruct three-dimensional (3D) mental picture of anatomy and pathology based on imaging studies. This aids in determining an approach, to achieve adequate exposure for complete tumor clearance and avoid complications.

The author emphasizes on implementing a dissection setup as close to the actual skull base operating room in order to develop fixed protocols in skull base surgery. He also suggests performing cadaveric dissection in team of two surgeons, as in many of the approaches, a two-surgeon bi-nostril technique is described. This two-surgeon team would have one surgeon who holds the endoscope to maintain a constant yet dynamic view and other would operate bimanually. It is of vital importance that both the surgeons have adequate knowledge of endoscopic anatomy and are equally oriented to the field. This would help the team develop much required coordination that is pivotal in skull base surgery.

This book describes various endonasal endoscopic approaches to access the entire ventral skull base extending from the frontal sinus anteriorly to the second cervical vertebra posteriorly and laterally till the infratemporal fossae on both the sides. The approaches are classified in the planes along the long axis of the various anatomical regions they provide access to.

General Principles

It is of paramount importance to understand that endoscopic skull base surgery is a deeply invasive procedure performed through the natural nasal ostium. Adherence to certain principles during skull base surgery facilitates to form surgical protocols to achieve predictable outcomes and avoid complications.

It is through collaborative efforts of various subspecialties that over the past two decades there has been a revolutionary advancement in ventral skull base (VSB) surgery. A well-organized team of the otorhinolaryngologist, neurosurgeon, anesthetist, endocrinologist, intensivist, and radiologist should work in unison to plan, perform, and achieve superior outcomes in VSB surgery.

It is essential for a surgeon to have a preoperative 3D orientation of the lesion and the most appropriate approach to be implemented for a safe and maximal resection of the skull base pathology. Preoperative planning of approach and reconstruction helps predict vital neurovascular structures that may be encountered, thus avoiding complications. This habit should be inculcated by a dissectors/trainees in early part of their skull base career.

There are some fundamental differences in basic operative etiquettes of functional endoscopic sinus surgery (FESS) and endoscopic VSB surgery. Dissection in FESS aims at restoring function of the mucociliary transport of the nose and paranasal sinuses and is rather a "mucosa preserving" procedure. Dissection during nasal phase in VSB surgery is primarily directed toward achieving maximal exposure for optimal access. The mucosa of the concerned sinus in the surgical trajectory is stripped off to expose the underlying bone. This avoids mucosal bleed while performing further steps, promotes graft uptake, and also prevents mucocele formation in the postoperative period. The operative concept is to be more radical in the nasal extradural phase and delicate and cautious during the intradural part of dissection (microdissection).

Wide exposure is obtained in the extradural part of VSB dissections. This is achieved by a partial resection of the middle turbinate on the right side with bilateral posterior ethmoidectomies. A cavity and half exposure is obtained. ("One and half" cavity exposure indicates one side nasal cavity and sphenoid sinus for instrumentation and another half created by posterior ethmoidectomy for parking the 4-mm endoscope.) This exposure is almost always done in VSB approaches.

A bi-nostril four-handed approach is an essential prerequisite for endoscopic VBS surgery for two main reasons. First, a bimanual microdissection enhances the surgeon's dexterity and maneuverability in critical areas as it utilizes a bi-nostril corridor and two instruments simultaneously. Second, clear dynamic views can be provided (a panned-out view for orientation and close-up view around critical structures) irrespective of the position of the instruments. Another advantage of the four-handed approach is the reduced frequency of soiling of the telescope that the co-surgeon/dissector can clear with irrigations. This minimizes surgeon's fatigue.

While performing a bimanual dissection, it is essential that surgeons have the access to both the nasal cavities through each of the nostrils. Thereby a posterior septectomy or a septal window is a prerequisite for such a bi-nostril access (**Fig. 5.1**).

It is advisable that while performing bimanual dissection, the assistant surgeon introduces the scope in the superior part of the right nostril. A nasal suction canula

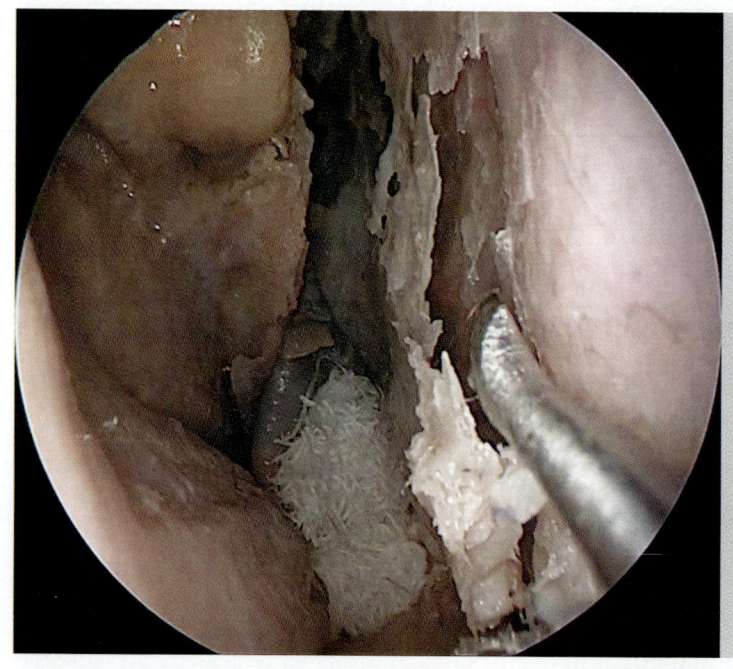

Fig. 5.1 Endoscopic image showing posterior septectomy being performed from the right side. The bony cartilaginous junction is separated after elevating the Hadad nasoseptal flap, and posterior bony part of the septum with appropriate part of the septum is removed. The mucoperichondrium on the other side is either removed or raised as a flap.

Tips and Tricks in Ventral Skull Base Dissection

that is held by the surgeon in his/her left hand is now introduced in the lower part of the nasal aperture on this side. The surgeon holds the primary/operating instrument in the right hand, and it is introduced in the left nostril (**Fig. 5.2**). A blunt nontraumatic suction in the surgeon's left hand can be used as a yardstick for depth perception and also for tissue retraction during the dissection of fibrous or solid tumors.

Skull base surgery is a finely coordinated effort, and the members of the two-surgeon team should understand others' requirements, capabilities, and limitations. It is necessary to maintain a constant team to perform dissections and surgeries comfortably (**Fig. 5.3**).

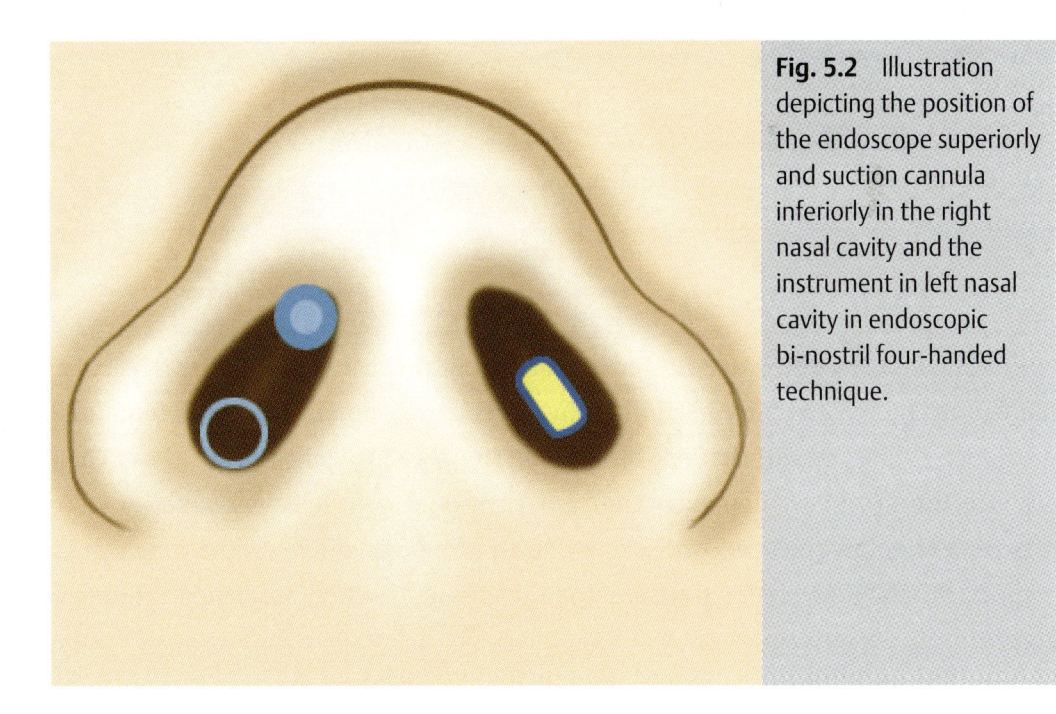

Fig. 5.2 Illustration depicting the position of the endoscope superiorly and suction cannula inferiorly in the right nasal cavity and the instrument in left nasal cavity in endoscopic bi-nostril four-handed technique.

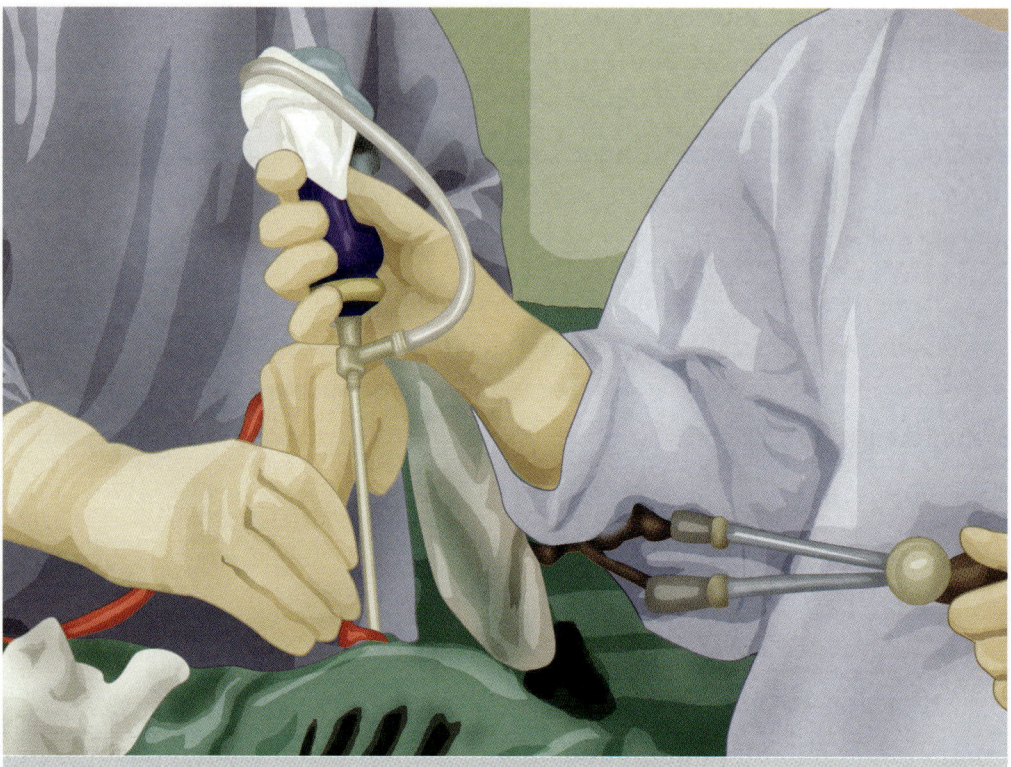

Fig. 5.3 Illustration depicting bi-nostril four-handed technique.

VSB surgery needs a dedicated set of highly precise instruments. Particular maneuvers are persistently performed by specific instruments. When a bimanual dissection is performed, the instruments or the telescope should not cross each other restricting their independent movement. It is prudent to have a superior view (instrument below the telescope) except for in some unavoidable situation such as a suprasellar dissections or transnasal craniectomy or when an angled telescope is used.

Tips and Tricks in Ventral Skull Base Dissection

Finally, it is through numerous dissection and practice sessions that a surgeon acquires skills in endoscopic skull base surgery. It enables the surgeon to develop attitude, coordination, temperament, and precision in this field. Cadaveric dissections are essential prerequisites as the surgeon ascends up along the levels of VSB surgery (**Fig. 5.4**).

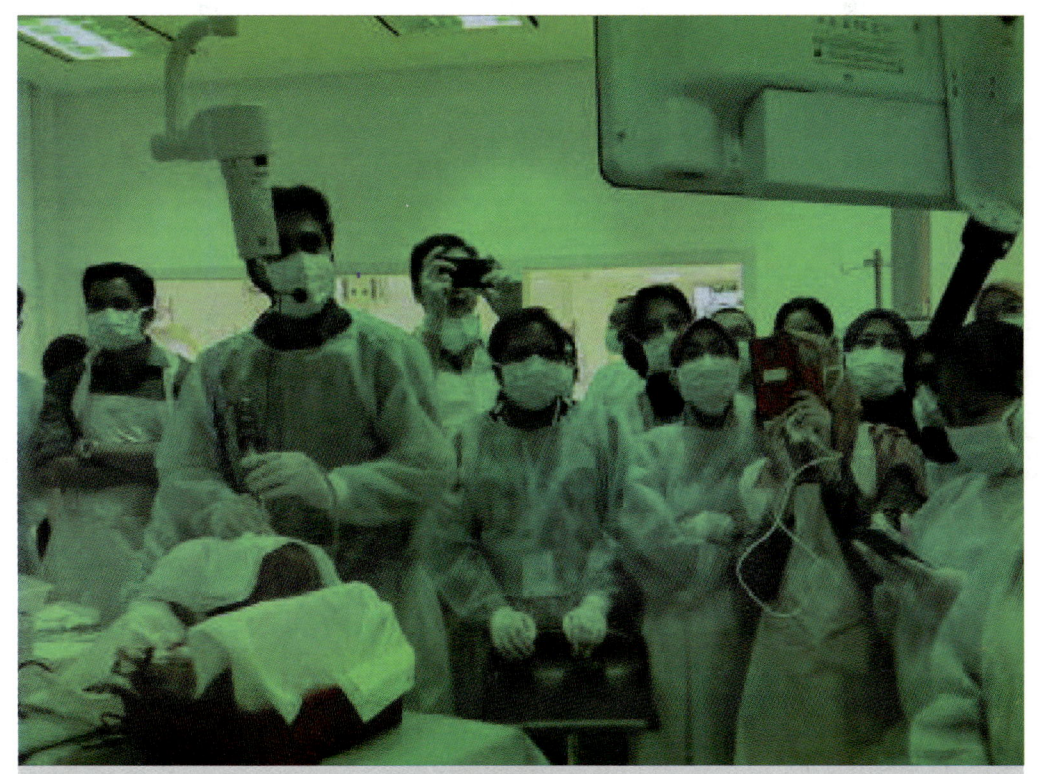

Fig. 5.4 Author briefing over a cadaveric dissection.

06 Dissection of Vascularized Pedicled Flaps in Ventral Skull Base Reconstruction

Narayanan Janakiram, Dharambir S. Sethi, Onkar K. Deshmukh, and Arvindh K. Gananathan

- § Introduction 85
- § Hadad Flap (Video 5) 86
- § Inferior Turbinate Flap (Video 6) 91
- § Middle Turbinate Flap 96
- § Pericranial Flap 96

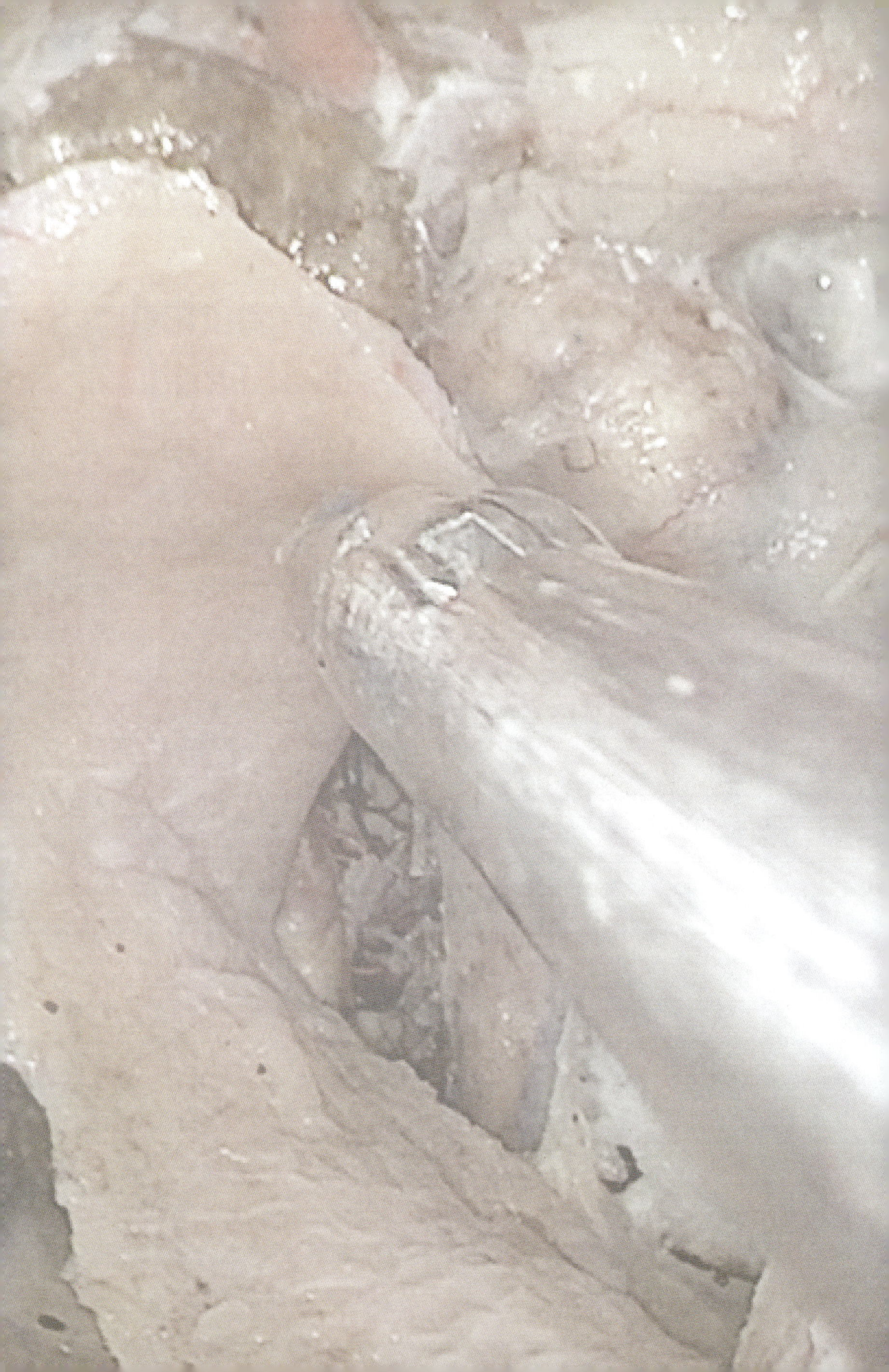

Introduction

Over the last few decades, advancements in instrumentation, technique, and expertise have revolutionized endoscopic endonasal skull-base surgery. With bigger and deep-seated tumors being extirpated through the endoscopic route, the size of the defect also increases. A thorough knowledge of reconstructive techniques is essential for ensuring adequate closure and thus avoiding postoperative complications.

The goals of skull-base reconstruction are to primarily create a watertight barrier between the cranial cavity and sinonasal tract, obliterate dead space created by the tumor removal, and to protect neurovascular structures. It is of paramount importance that the reconstruction achieves complete separation of the cranial and nasal cavities. Incomplete closures of skull-base defects are associated with persistent cerebrospinal fluid (CSF) leak and potential risk of meningitis, which can be catastrophic and potentially fatal in the postoperative period.

As endoscopic reconstruction ventral skull-base defects may involve use of tissues from the nasal cavity itself, it is prudent to plan reconstruction prior to commencement of tumor removal. The factors that determine the type of reconstruction include the size, location and the suspected histopathology of the tumor, presence of intraoperative CSF leak, and if so, whether or not it is a high-flow leak, etc.

There is a spectrum of reconstructive techniques involving combinations of free tissue grafts, vascularized pedicled flaps, and allogenic materials in a multilayered fashion. Literature suggests that the use of vascularized pedicled flaps in reconstruction of skull-base defects results in superior surgical outcomes by achieving postoperative CSF leak below 5%.[1-3]

Vascularized nasal mucosa is an important resource for skull-base reconstruction. While free tissue grafts cover the defect and act as a template for mucosalization, the pedicled flaps close the defect and integrate with the nasal mucosa surrounding the free edge of the flap. In case of an intraoperative CSF leak, ability of the skull-base surgeon to raise a local pedicled flap in primary or a revision case is pivotal to avoid postoperative leaks.

During cadaveric dissection, the dissectors should familiarize themselves with endoscopic techniques to raise various endonasal vascularized flaps (**Table 6.1**). These include primarily the nasoseptal Hadad flap with its modifications and others like the inferior turbinate flap, the anterior ethmoidal flap, the pericranial flap, and the temporoparietal flap.

Hadad Flap (Video 5)

The nasoseptal flap (Hadad–Bassagasteguy flap [HBF]) is a vascularized pedicle flap of nasal septum which gets its supply from the nasoseptal artery, a branch of sphenopalatine artery (**Fig. 6.1**). HBF is used to repair defects of anterior, middle, clival, and parasellar region. HBF was first described in 2006 by Hadad et al and was named Hadad–Bassagasteguy flap. This has significantly reduced the incidence of CSF leak postoperatively.[1-6]

Table 6.1 Locoregional vascularized flaps in endoscopic skull-base reconstruction

Intranasal vascularized flaps
1. Nasoseptal Hadad flap
2. Inferior turbinate flap
3. Middle turbinate flap
Extranasal vascularized flaps
1. Pericranial flap
2. Temporoparietal flap

Dissection of Vascularized Pedicled Flaps

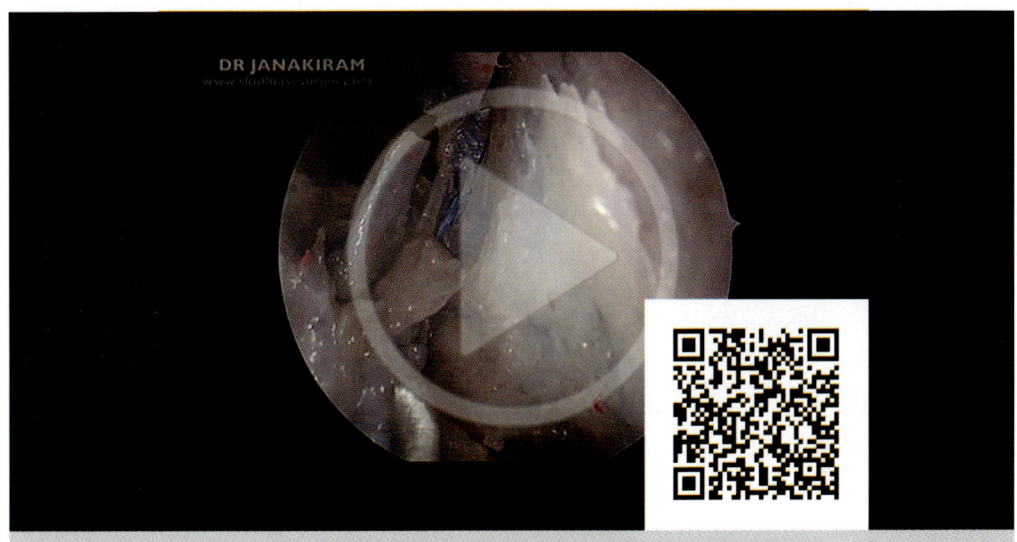

Video 5 Hadad flap. https://www.thieme.de/de/q.htm?p=opn/tp/388257077/9789388257060_c001_v005&t=video

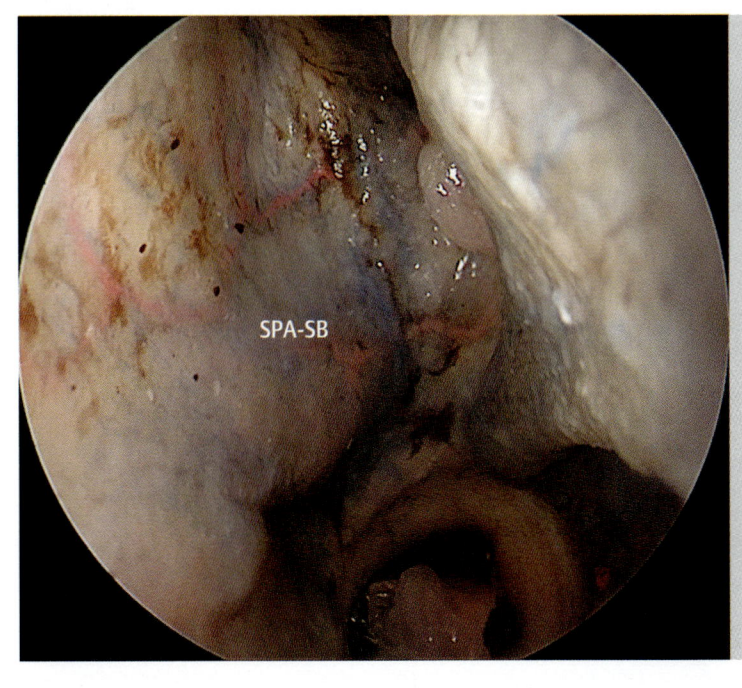

Fig. 6.1 Endoscopic image showing septal branch of SPA. SPA-SB, septal branch of sphenopalatine artery.

The dissection of HBF starts with lateralization of inferior turbinate, partial resection of middle turbinate. Usually flap is taken on the right side or the side of flap is determined by the lesions. If the lesion is present in lateral to pterygoid, we have to drill on pterygoid which will compromise the vascularity of the flap for which opposite side HBF is taken.

Two horizontal incisions are made in the coronal plane parallel to each other; superior incision is made from below the sphenoid OS extending 1 to 2 cm below the level of superior part of septum. The inferior incision is made from posterior choana along the free edge of posterior septum extended along the maxillary crest. The vertical incision is made at the mucocutaneous junction joining the horizontal incisions. The elevation of the flap starts anteriorly with Cottle's elevator; posteriorly the dissection is complete after elevating from the anterior face of sphenoid sinus saving the vascular pedicle. In case of large defects, we can take an extended Hadad flap which includes the mucoperiosteum of floor of nose (**Fig. 6.2**).

The nasoseptal rescue flap is indicated in case where CSF leak is possible but most likely to happen. In this technique, the pedicle of the HBF is protected without raising the entire flap.[7] The initial steps are similar to HBF—the exposure and two horizontal incisions extending till the anterior end of the middle turbinate followed by elevation.

A ball probe is used to elevate till the mucoperichondrium. The entire posterior aspect of the flap elevation is done till anterior face of sphenoid sinus; thus transposing the flap downwards. The ipsilateral dissection of the sphenoid can then be done without injuring the pedicle without raising the entire flap (**Fig. 6.3**).

Dissection of Vascularized Pedicled Flaps

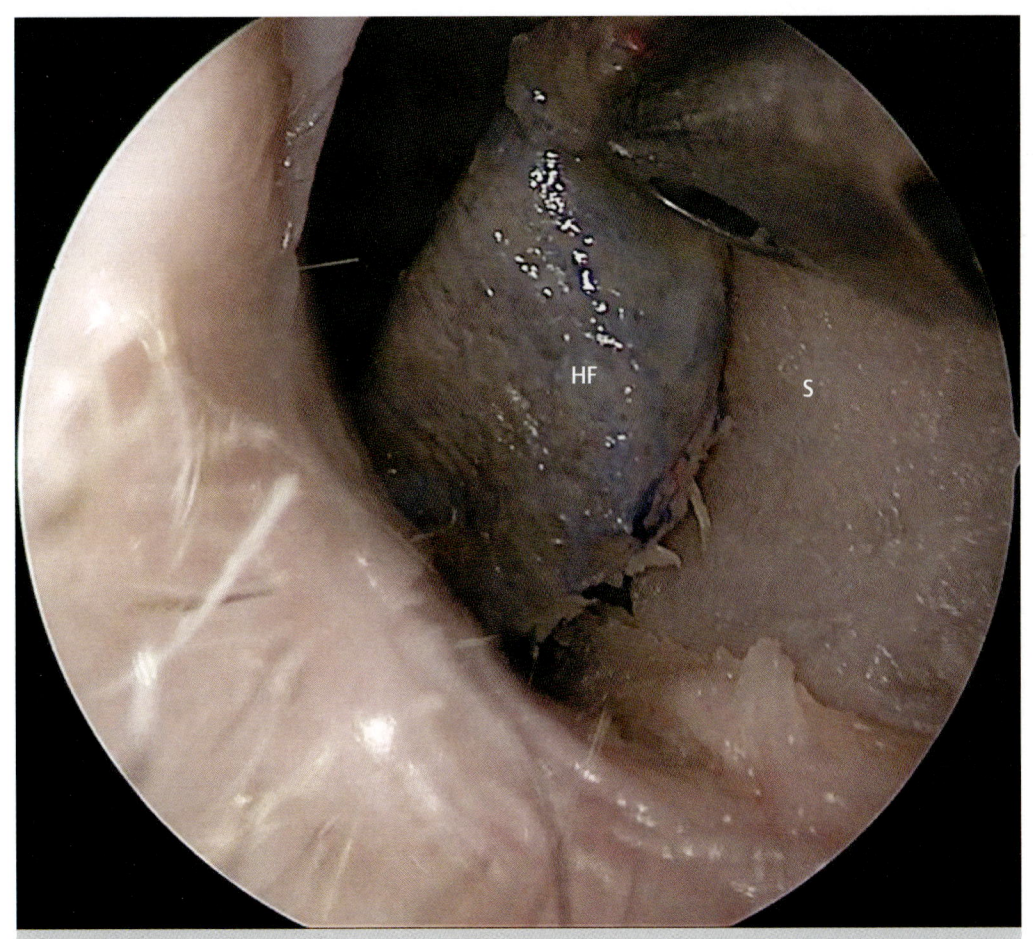

Fig. 6.2 Endoscopic image showing raising the Hadad-Bassagasteguy flap. HF, Hadad flap; S, septum.

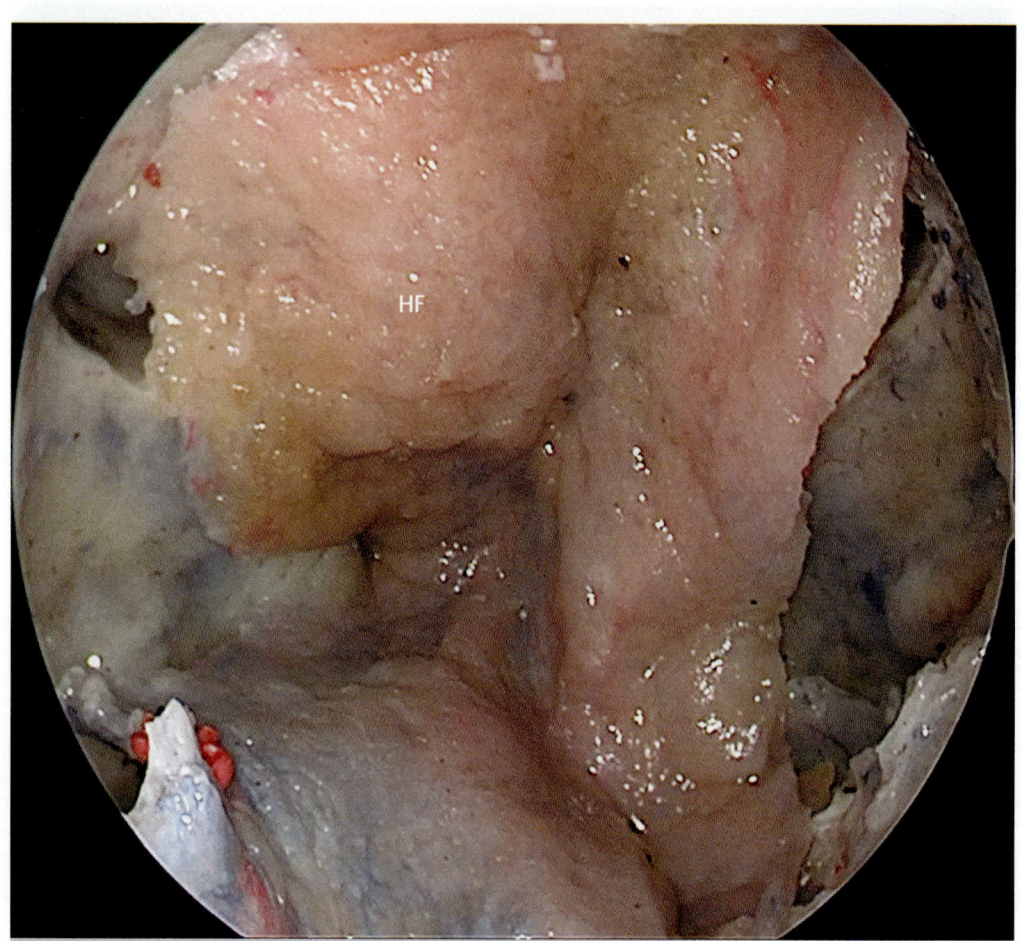

Fig. 6.3 Endoscopic image showing placement of the Hadad-Bassagasteguy flap for covering the anterior skull base defect. HF, Hadad flap.

Inferior Turbinate Flap (Video 6)

In revision cases, where the nasoseptal HBF has already been used or a septectomy has been performed, the inferior turbinate flap is a requisite alternative for reconstruction. The inferior turbinate is supplied by a terminal branch of the posterior lateral nasal artery which is indeed a branch of sphenopalatine artery.[8] The pedicle enters the inferior turbinate at the superior aspect of its lateral attachment 1.2 to 1.5 cm from its posterior end.

To harvest the inferior turbinate flap, the inferior turbinate is medialized to facilitate access to its medial as well as the lateral surfaces. An incision in the horizontal plane commencing at the superior insertion of middle turbinate is continued in the posteroanterior direction (**Fig. 6.4**). Now a vertical incision is taken starting from the superior incision, sloping around the contour of the head of the inferior turbinate and onto the inferior meatus (**Fig. 6.5**). The mucosal flap is elevated from the lateral wall of the nose along the middle meatal area and medial surface of the inferior turbinate; the mucosa over the lateral surface may also be included, if a larger defect is to be reconstructed. A Cottle's elevator is used to elevate the flap in subperiosteal plane. Posteriorly, the flap is elevated up to its pedicle. When the mucosa over the floor of the nasal cavity is included along with that over the lateral surface of the inferior turbinate, the resultant flap is termed as extended inferior turbinate flap (**Fig. 6.6**).

Though not as versatile as the HBF owing to a smaller arc of rotation, ipsilateral inferior turbinate flap are commonly used to reconstruct sphenoidal roof defects and clival defects, especially in revision cases (**Fig. 6.7**).

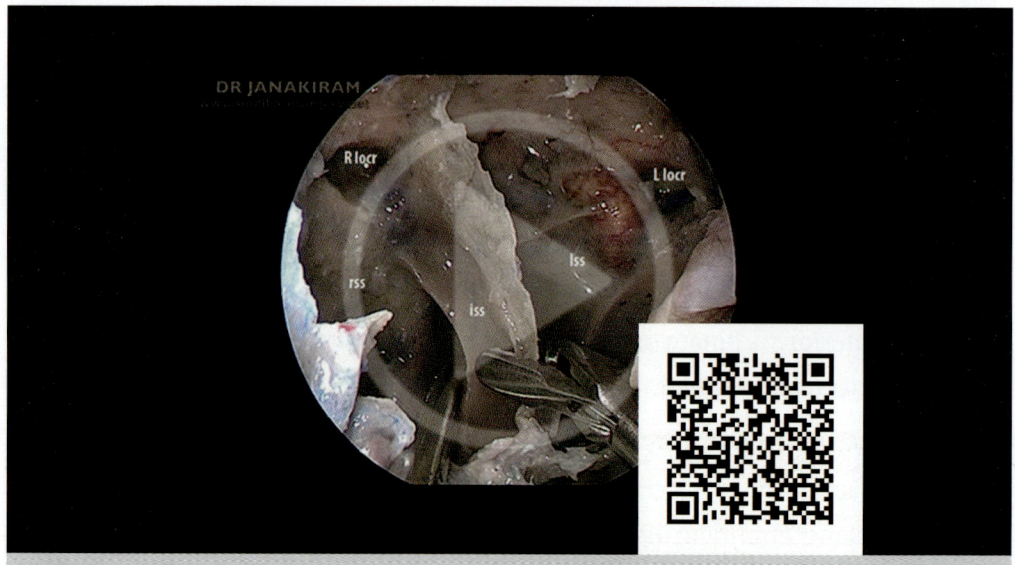

Video 6 Inferior turbinate flap (lateral nasal wall flap). https://www.thieme.de/de/q.htm?p=opn/tp/388257077/9789388257060_c001_v006&t=video

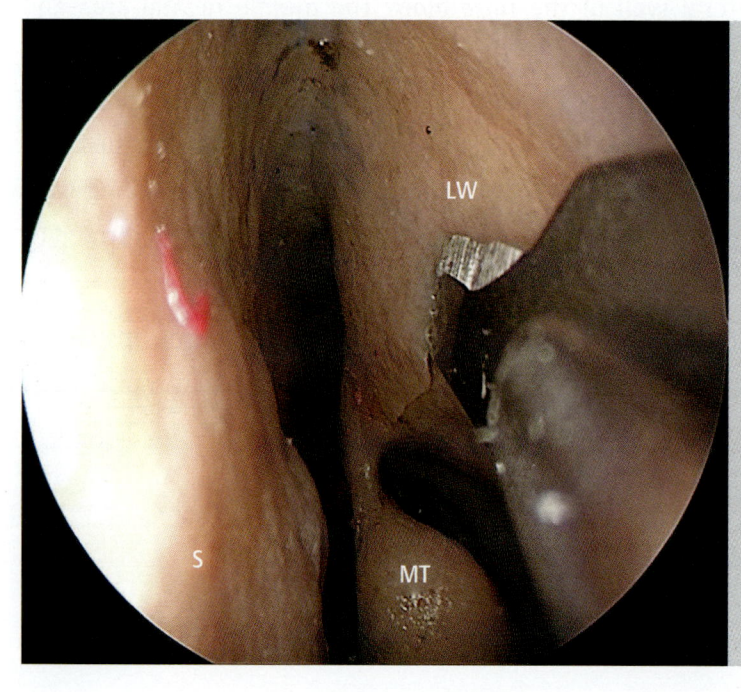

Fig. 6.4 Endoscopic image showing horizontal incision for the inferior turbinate flap. LW, lateral wall; MT, middle turbinate; S, septum.

Dissection of Vascularized Pedicled Flaps

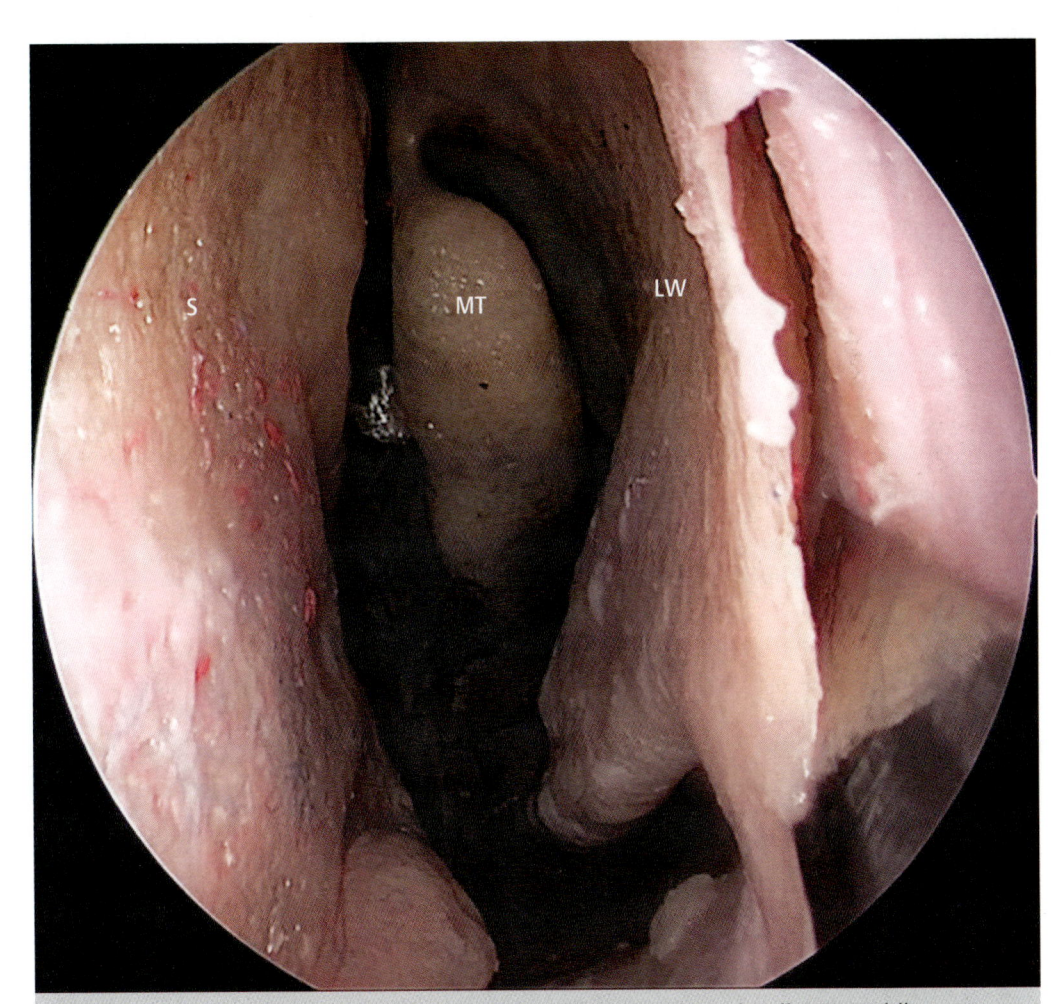

Fig. 6.5 Endoscopic image showing anterior incision. LW, lateral wall; MT, middle turbinate; S, septum.

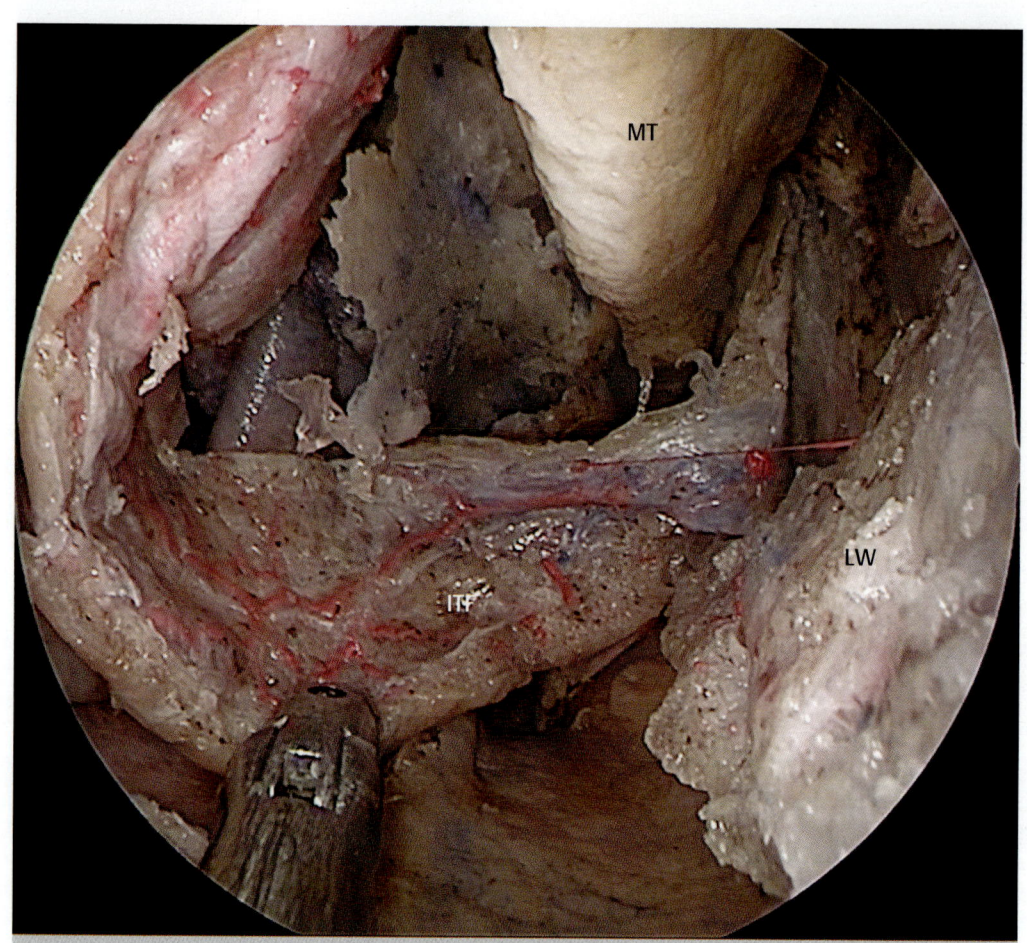

Fig. 6.6 Endoscopic image showing raising inferior turbinate flap. ITF, inferior turbinate flap; LW, lateral wall of the nasal cavity; MT, middle turbinate.

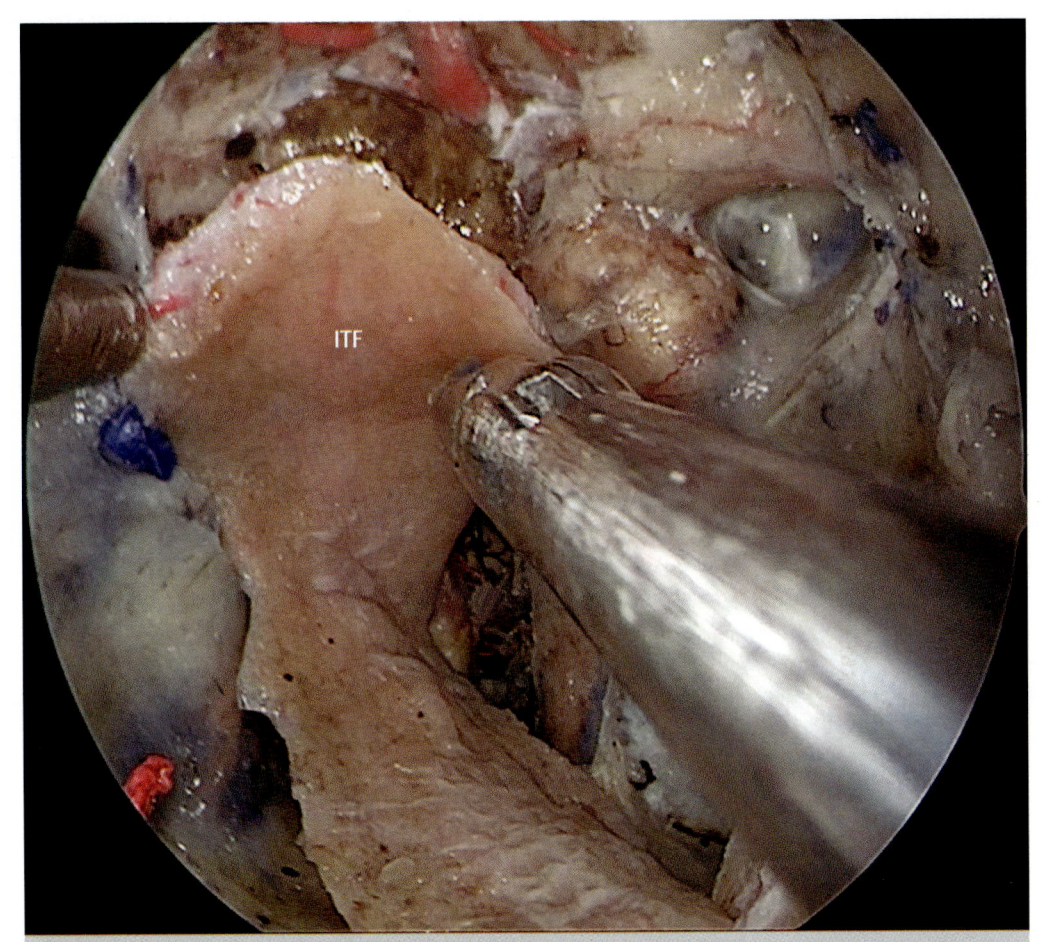

Fig. 6.7 Endoscopic image showing placement of the flap. ITF, inferior turbinate flap.

Middle Turbinate Flap

Middle turbinate flap has similar indications than that of the inferior turbinate flap. The posterior nasal artery gives a branch to the middle turbinate as it does to the inferior turbinate.[8] This flap is used for the reconstruction of defects in fovea, sella, and planum. Owing to its small surface, this flap has very limited applications.

This flap is avoided when the middle turbinate has anatomical variations like concha bullosa or a paradoxical curvature or is unstable at its attachment.

A vertical incision is given through the mucosa of the middle turbinate anteriorly. This is followed by an incision over the superomedial aspect of the middle turbinate posteriorly till the pedicle. The mucosa over the medial aspect is then elevated with a Cottle's elevator. The bone of the middle turbinate is taken out part by part and another horizontal incision is given in the axilla proceeding in the dorsal direction. Once the turbinate is separated from its attachment, the medial and lateral mucosal surfaces of the middle turbinate are opened and separated from each other. The pedicle is raised posteriorly till the sphenopalatine foramen area (**Fig. 6.8**). Caution should be exercised not to damage the attachment of the turbinate to the lamellae of the cribriform plate.

Pericranial Flap

The main intent of using the pericranial flap is to cover large defects and separate the sinonasal track from intracranial space with a vascularized tissue in cases where HBF is not available.[9] The HBF is compromised and pericranial flap serves as a good source of reconstruction. In-depth knowledge of the vascular supply of the flap is necessary for dissection. The flap is supplied by the supraorbital and supratrochlear artery; superficial branches from these arteries will course into the

Dissection of Vascularized Pedicled Flaps

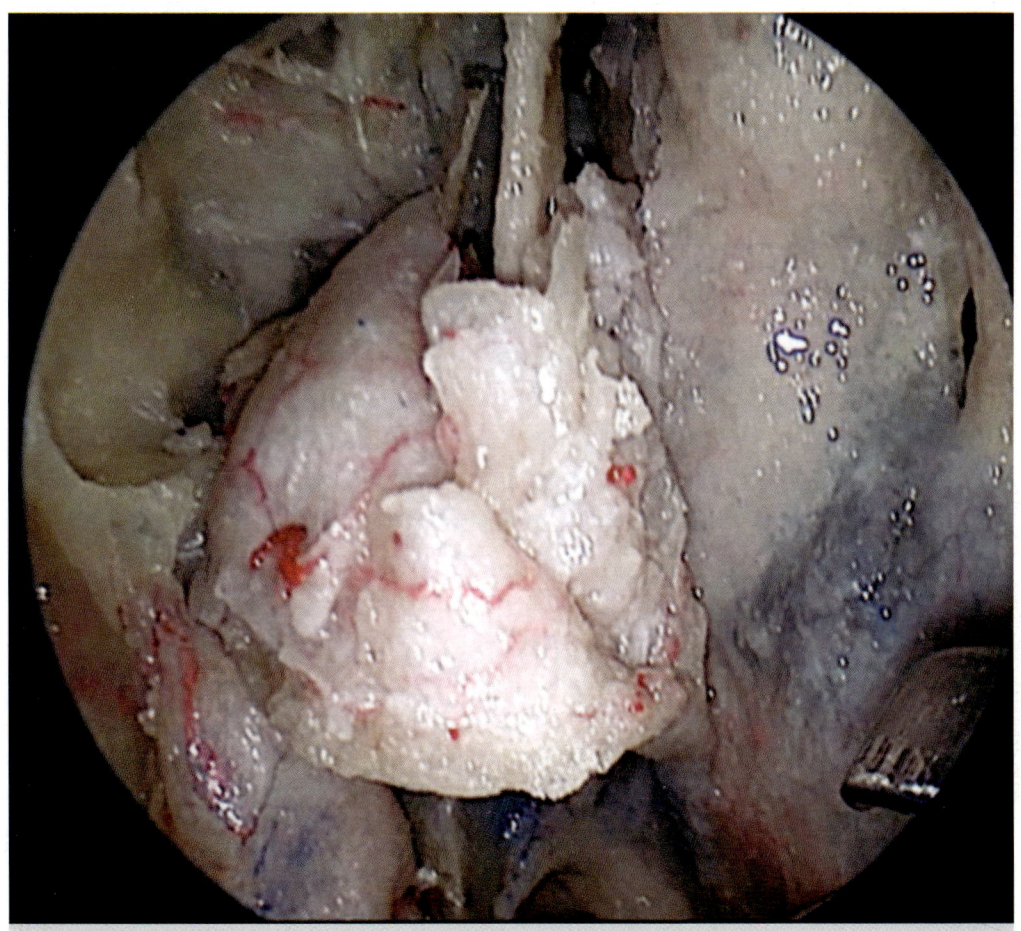

Fig. 6.8 Endoscopic image showing middle turbinate flap.

galea and frontalis muscle, deep branch from which will supply the pericranium. Deep branch may exit 1 cm above the exit point of supraorbital and supratrochlear foramen so one should keep in mind dissecting beyond this level.

At the author's center, dissection starts with a bicoronal incision from 1 cm anterior to the tragus terminates above the zygomatic arch ending on the opposite side same area (**Fig. 6.9**). The incision is deep through the galea and the loose areolar tissue plane is identified and the flap is elevated anteriorly till the supra orbital rim on both sides (**Fig. 6.10**). The incision on the pericranial flap extends from 3 cm pedicle from supraorbital rim going laterally along the temporal line extending posteriorly till the bicoronal incision. Then the incision progresses toward the midline scalp and then toward the midline to the glabella (**Fig. 6.11**). The elevation of the pericranial flap is done using elevator. Elevation is done till the supraorbital rim (**Fig. 6.12**). After harvesting the pericranial flap, it has to be transposed to the nasal cavity for which osteotomies is performed in the nasion from medial canthus to medial cantus protecting the medial canthal ligament. The osteotomies created are around 1 to 1.5 cm wide and 4 mm high. The dissected pericranial flap is then transposed into the nasal cavity. The Draf III procedure is done prior to these steps and the flap is brought through the middle of the frontal sinus floor to cover the dural defect after removal of tumor.

Over the past two decades, with expansion in access and extent of endonasal endoscopic corridors, the demand for vascularized reconstructive option also increases. However, much like other centers, at the authors' center too, the nasoseptal HBF still remains the primary choice for reconstruction. This is attributed to its expanded paddle and long length of the pedicle as well as better arc of rotation. Other flaps are considered in revision cases or otherwise, where the nasoseptal flap is not available. Depending on the defect size and location either inferior turbinate flap or a pericranial flap is raised at the authors' center. The pericranial flap is chosen for a larger or a longer defect in revision cases. The middle turbinate flap is rarely used. An anterior ethmoidal flap is also seldom used to reduce the cicatrisational narrowing of the Draf III cavity.

Dissection of Vascularized Pedicled Flaps

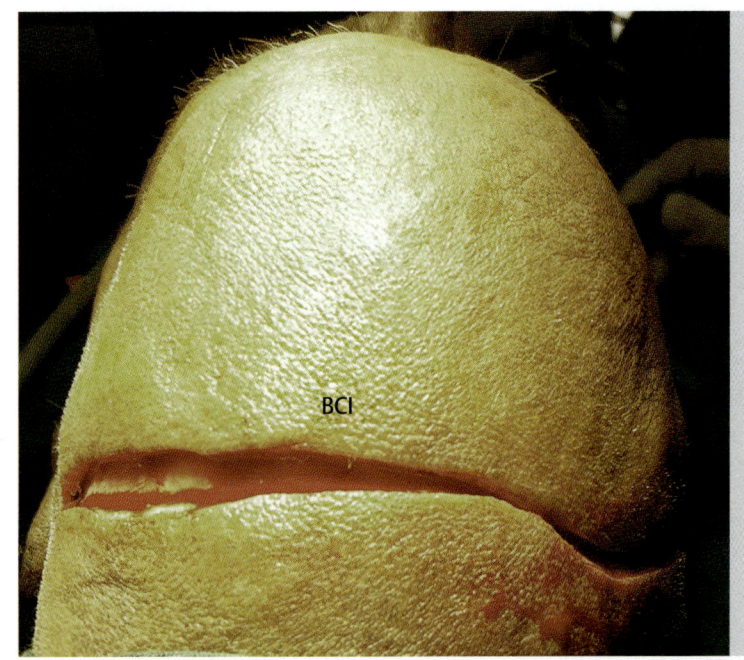

Fig. 6.9 Image showing the incision for raising the flap. BCI, bicoronal incision.

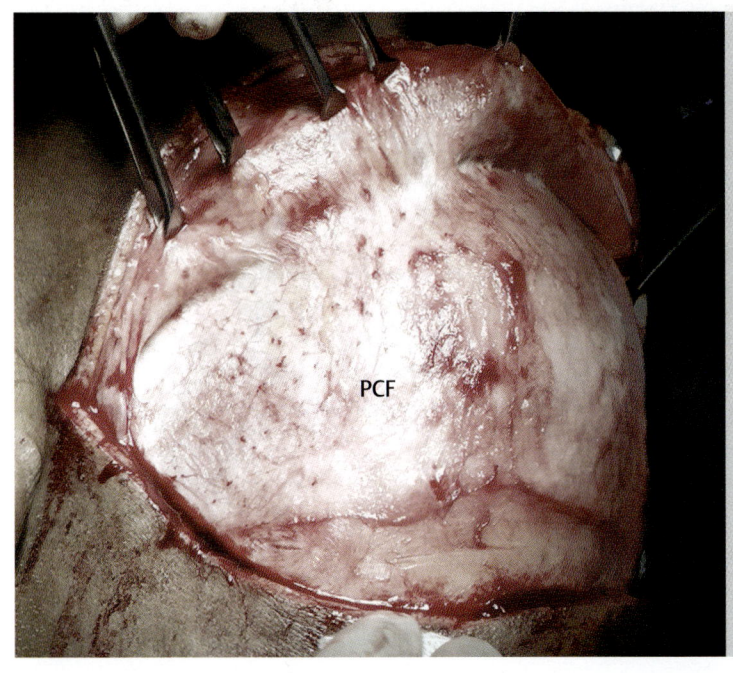

Fig. 6.10 Image showing raising of the galea aponeurotica. PCF, pericranial flap.

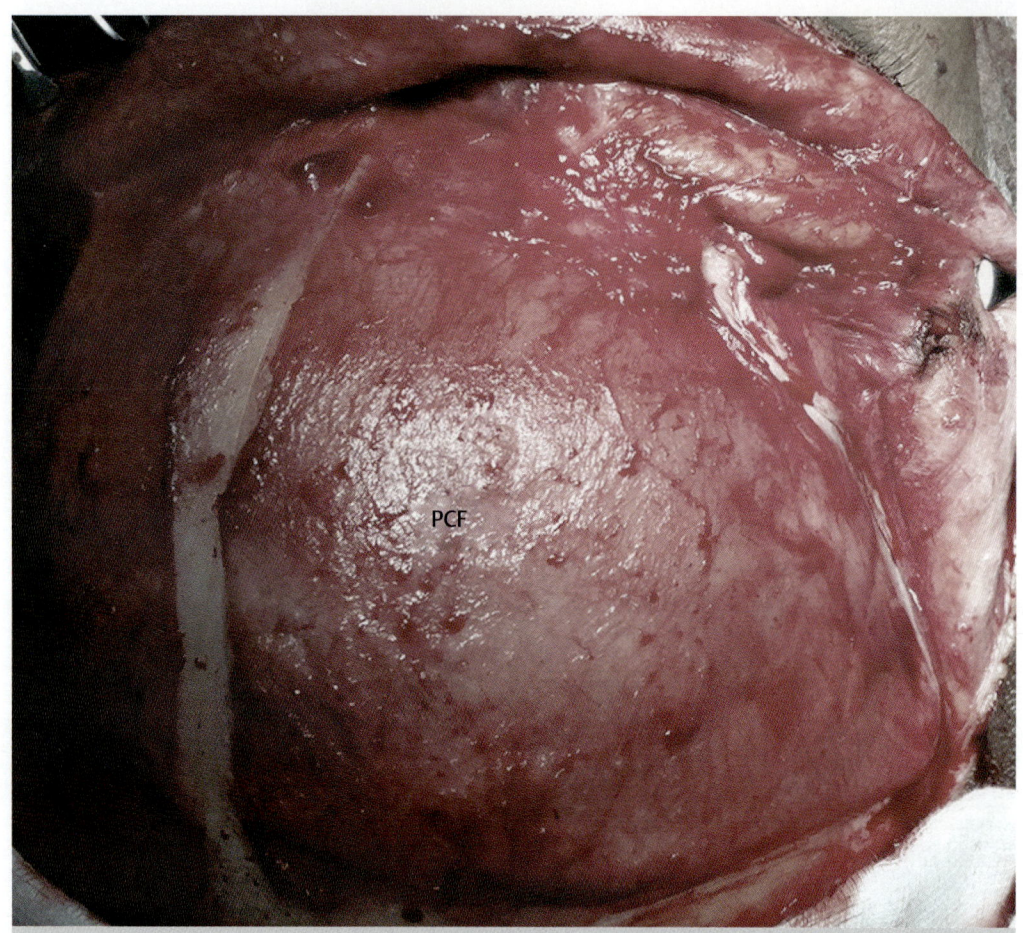

Fig. 6.11 Image showing incision on the pericranium. PCF, pericranial flap.

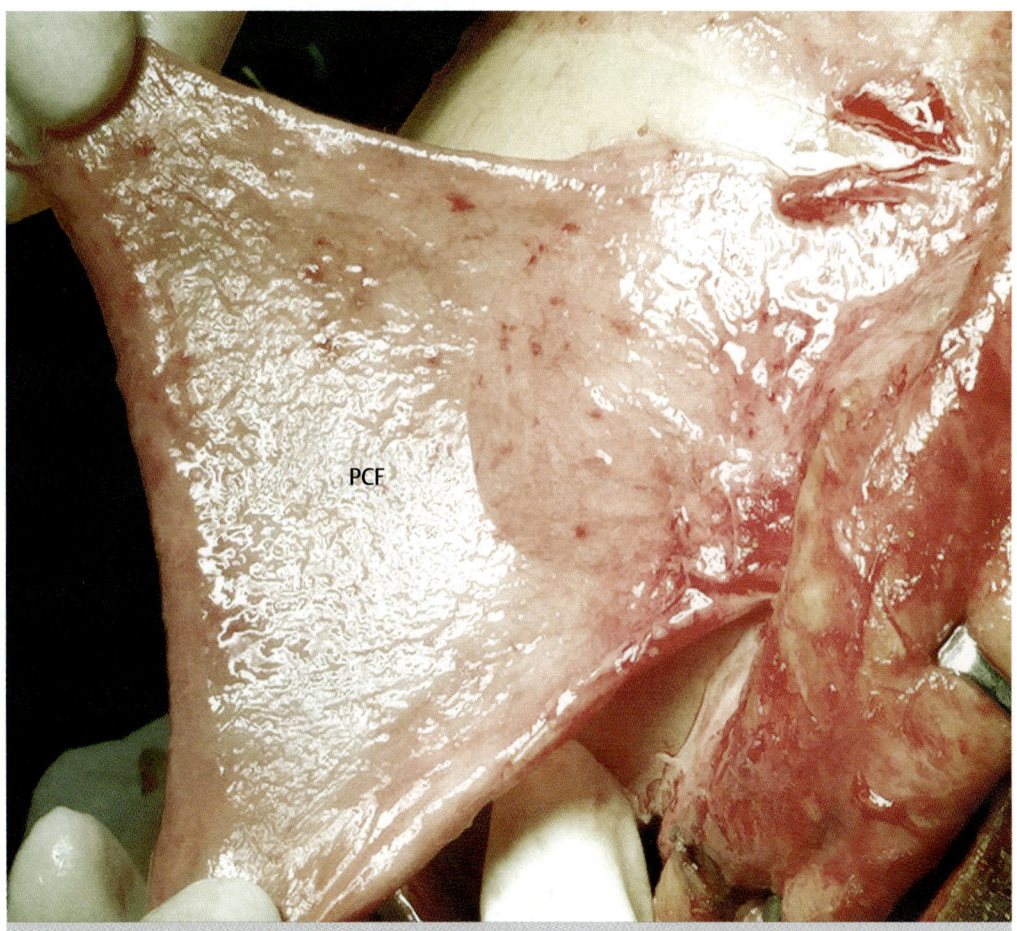

Fig. 6.12 Image showing the harvested pericranial flap. PCF, pericranial flap.

With technical expertise and thoughtful planning of the vascularized reconstructive option, there is significant reduction in the postoperative complication rate in endoscopic skull-base surgery. A trainee skull-base surgeon should be at least confident in raising a nasoseptal flap in situations where the reconstructive need be such. Other flaps can be raised in subsequently as knowledge, technique, and expertise graduate along the learning curve.

References

1. Hadad G, Bassagasteguy L, Carrau RL, et al. A novel reconstructive technique after endoscopic expanded endonasal approaches: vascular pedicle nasoseptal flap. Laryngoscope 2006;116(10):1882–1886

2. Kassam AB, Thomas A, Carrau RL, et al. Endoscopic reconstruction of the cranial base using a pedicled nasoseptal flap. Neurosurgery 2008;63(1, Suppl 1):ONS44–ONS52, discussion ONS52–ONS53

3. Kassam AB, Prevedello DM, Carrau RL, et al. Endoscopic endonasal skull base surgery: analysis of complications in the authors' initial 800 patients. J Neurosurg 2011;114(6):1544–1568

4. White DR, Dubin MG, Senior BA. Endoscopic repair of cerebrospinal fluid leaks after neurosurgical procedures. Am J Otolaryngol 2003;24(4):213–216

5. Leong JL, Citardi MJ, Batra PS. Reconstruction of skull base defects after minimally invasive endoscopic resection of anterior skull base neoplasms. Am J Rhinol 2006; 20(5):476–482

6. Esposito F, Dusick JR, Fatemi N, Kelly DF. Graded repair of cranial base defects and cerebrospinal fluid leaks in transsphenoidal surgery. Neurosurgery 2007; 60(4, Suppl 2):295–303, discussion 303–304

7. Rivera-Serrano CM, Snyderman CH, Gardner P, et al. Nasoseptal "rescue" flap: a novel modification of the nasoseptal flap technique for pituitary surgery. Laryngoscope 2011;121(5):990–993

8. Chakravarthi S, Gonen L, Monroy-Sosa A, Khalili S, Kassam A. Endoscopic endonasal reconstructive methods to the anterior skull base. Semin Plast Surg 2017;31(4): 203–213

9. Patel MR, Shah RN, Snyderman CH, et al. Pericranial flap for endoscopic anterior skull-base reconstruction: clinical outcomes and radioanatomic analysis of preoperative planning. Neurosurgery 2010;66(3):506–512, discussion 512

07 Endoscopic Approaches in Sagittal Plane

Narayanan Janakiram, Dharambir S. Sethi, Arvindh K. Gananathan, and Onkar K. Deshmukh

- § Introduction 107
- § Transfrontal Approach 107
- § Endoscopic Transnasal Craniectomy Approach 116
- § Endoscopic Transnasal Transsphenoidal Approaches 122
- § Nasal Phase 128
- § Trans-sellar Approach (Video 10) 133
- § Transtuberculum Approach (Video 10) 136
- § Transplanum Approach 136
- § Transclival Approach (Videos 11 and 12) 141

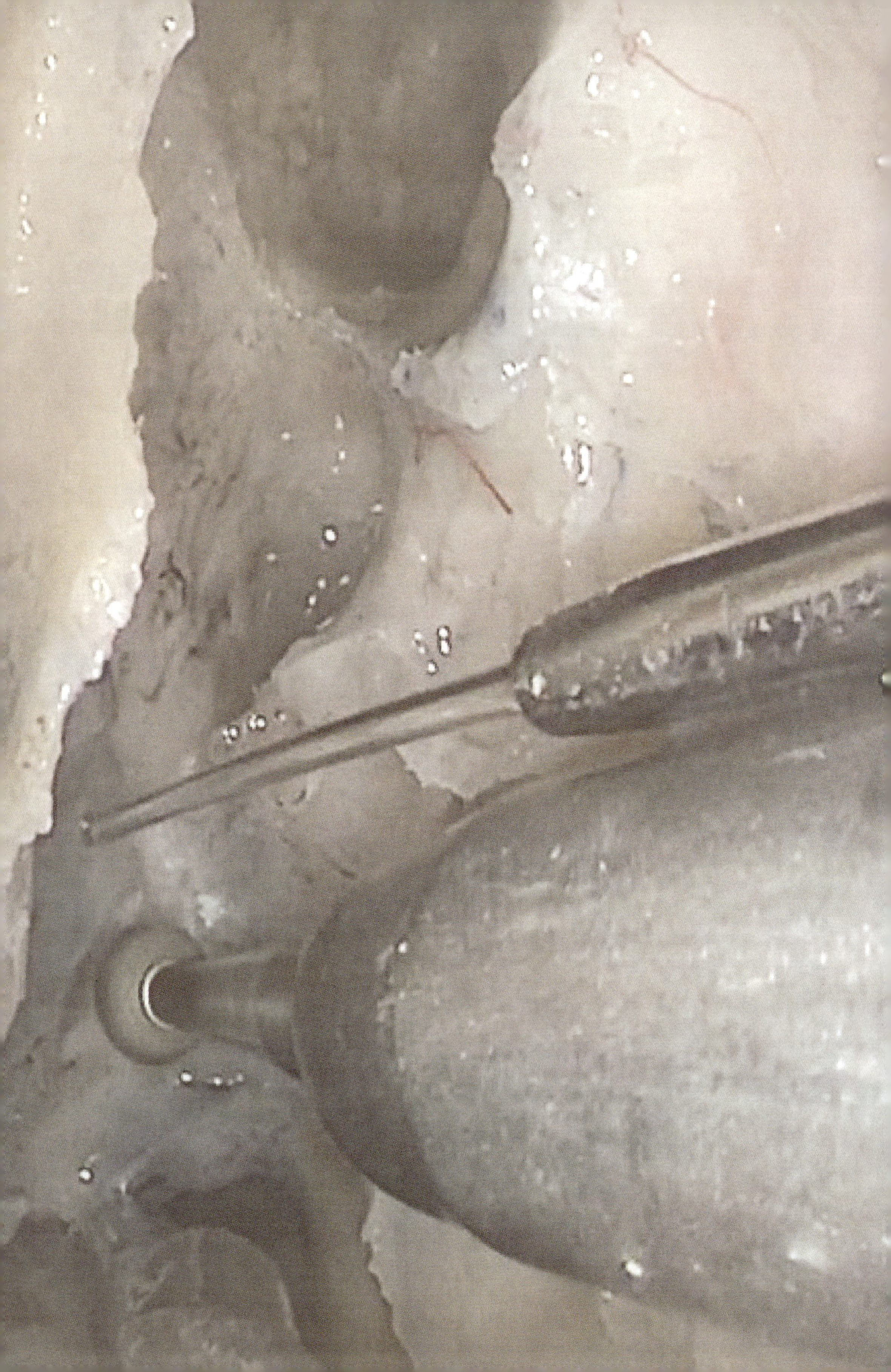

Introduction

This chapter elaborates approaches to anatomical subunits along the midline anteroposterior plane. This sagittal plane comprises the frontal sinus anteriorly extending through sphenoid sinus and clivus posteriorly. The various endoscopic approaches along this plane are mentioned in the **Table 4.1**.

Transfrontal Approach

The transfrontal approach provides access to the anterior most anatomical subunit of the ventral skull base in the sagittal plane. Pathologies extending into the frontal sinus laterally, lesions involving the frontal sinus or eroding the posterior table of frontal sinus, and posterior table fracture causing cerebrospinal fluid (CSF) leaks can be accessed with this approach. This approach is also adopted as an initial step in transcribriform approach. This procedure is also performed to provide a conduit for the pericranial flap that is introduced into the nasal cavity through a supraorbital bone window created at the medial brow region.[1]

Table 4.1 Approaches in sagittal plane

Endoscopic approaches in sagittal plane
• Transfrontal
• Transcribriform.
• Transsphenoidal 　○ Trans-sellar 　○ Transtuberculum 　○ Transplanum
• Transclival

This approach involves removal of superior part of the nasal septum, the floor of both the frontal sinuses, and connecting the two frontal sinuses to a single cavity that drains into the nose. This approach enables to skeletonize the entire ventral skull base.

Relevant Anatomy

The frontal sinus is a pneumatized space between the anterior and posterior tables of the frontal bone. Frontal sinuses on each side conform to a pyramidal shape and are separated by an interfrontal septum medially. It has four walls; the anterior and posterior walls are formed by the anterior and posterior tables of the frontal bone, respectively. The inferior or orbitonasal wall forms the floor of frontal sinus, and the medial wall is formed by the interfrontal septum.

The anterior wall or the thicker anterior table consists of a spongy bone lying between two thin lamellae of the cortical bone. It commences at the frontonasal suture line and ends superiorly at the frontal protuberance. It is covered by a very thick pericranium, frontalis muscle, subcutaneous tissue, and skin. This part of the pericranium is richly supplied by the supratrochlear vessels and is used a vascularized flap in skull base reconstructions.

The posterior wall separates the frontal sinus from the anterior cranial cavity and is in close contact with the dura of the frontal lobes. This wall is very thin and is prone to erosion by frontal pathologies.

The medial wall is a triangle-shaped intersinus septum, which separates the two frontal sinuses. At the level of the infundibulum of the frontal sinuses, it lies in the midline in its inferior part. This part is attached to the nasal spine of the frontal bone anteriorly, perpendicular plate of ethmoid inferiorly, and crista galli posteriorly. This wall can be pneumatized forming the interfrontal cell, which has a separate drainage.[2,3]

The orbitonasal or inferior wall is the part between the anterior and posterior tables inferiorly. This has a *lateral orbital part* and a *medial nasal part*. The *lateral* part lies between the orbit and frontal sinus. The anterior edge of this part forms the supraorbital rim. Medially the orbital part is delimited from the medial nasal part by the attachment of lamina papyracea and the lacrimal bone. The *medial* or *nasal* part of the inferior wall of the frontal sinus is a quadrangular plate of bone situated at a lower level to the orbital part and articulates medially, at its inferior aspect, with the vertical lateral lamella of the cribriform plate. The frontal sinus ostium is present in the most oblique portion of the of this wall, and depending on the ethmoid pneumatization, it can be a large opening extending till the orbital section that is referred as the "frontal bulla" or it may be a small slit-like ostium. Excessive thickness of the anterior part of the ostium results in formation of a tunnel-like structure opening in the frontal recess known as the *frontonasal duct.*

The frontal ostium opens in to the frontal recess. This passage is bounded by independent bony structures on all four sides. The medial wall is formed by the lateral lamella of the cribriform plate that continues as lateral surface of the sagittal part of the middle turbinate. The lateral lamella is a very thin plate of bone vulnerable to surgical trauma and iatrogenic CSF leak. The uncinate process depending on its attachment to the lamina or middle turbinate also forms a part of lateral or medial wall of the recess, respectively. The lamina papyracea forms the lateral wall of this recess. The ethmoidal bulla comprises the posterior wall, and agger nasi forms its anterior wall. Depending on their degrees of pneumatization, these cells, agger, and/or bulla may encroach upon the recess. The agger nasi is the anterior most ethmoidal pneumatization in the nasofrontal beak, formed by the thick ascending process of the maxilla.[4]

The cranial surface of the frontal bone anteriorly displays a medial sulcus, which contains the anterior part of the superior sagittal sinus. The edges of this sulcus unite to form the frontal crest. The frontal crest and edges of the sulcus give attachment to the falx cerebri. The frontal crest ends posteriorly in a small deficiency called as the *ethmoidal notch*. The orbital plates of the frontal bone extend beyond the orbital roof nasally on both sides to form lateral boundary of the ethmoidal notch. This orbital plate articulates with the lateral lamella of the cribriform plate that occupies the ethmoidal notch. The (vertical) lateral lamella and (horizontal) medial lamella form an angle at their junction that provides insertion to the sagittal part of the middle turbinate.

In the nasal cavity, the orbital plates of the frontal bone at their inferior aspect are integrated with the pneumatized ethmoidal labyrinth to form its roof or the fovea ethmoidalis. The orbital plate is continuous with the nasal part of the orbitonasal or inferior wall of the frontal sinus anteriorly. Posteriorly the orbital plate articulates with the lesser wing of the sphenoid. At both these margins of the orbital plate, transverse grooves are converted into anterior and posterior ethmoidal canals by articulation with the ethmoid bone. They transmit the anterior and posterior ethmoidal nerves and vessels. The fovea of the frontal sinus that includes the frontal ostium, lies anterior to the anterior ethmoidal artery, and is at a higher level to the ethmoidal fovea. The nasal part of the inferior wall of the frontal sinus that forms this fovea articulates with the nasal bone inferomedially and the ascending process of the maxilla inferolaterally. This ascending process or the frontal process of maxilla forms the nasofrontal beak and anterior to the axilla of middle turbinate covers the lacrimal sac.

Dissection (Video 7)

The surgery commences with a 0-degree endoscope and a two-handed uni-nostril approach. The mucosa over the frontal process of maxilla is debrided beginning anterior to the axilla of the middle turbinate (**Fig. 7.1**) proceeding superiorly and laterally all the way up to the roof of the nasal cavity, and maintaining the same anteroposterior plane, the blade is turned onto the septal mucosa denuding the septal cartilage. The denuded cartilage is incised, and a superior septectomy (~2 × 2 cm) is performed by incising the cartilage such that the posterior limit of the septectomy is at the level of the anterior end of the middle turbinate (**Fig. 7.2**). The lower margin of septectomy is approximately 0.5 cm below the lower border of the middle turbinate. The corresponding septal mucosa on the opposite side is debrided.

Endoscopic Approaches in Sagittal Plane

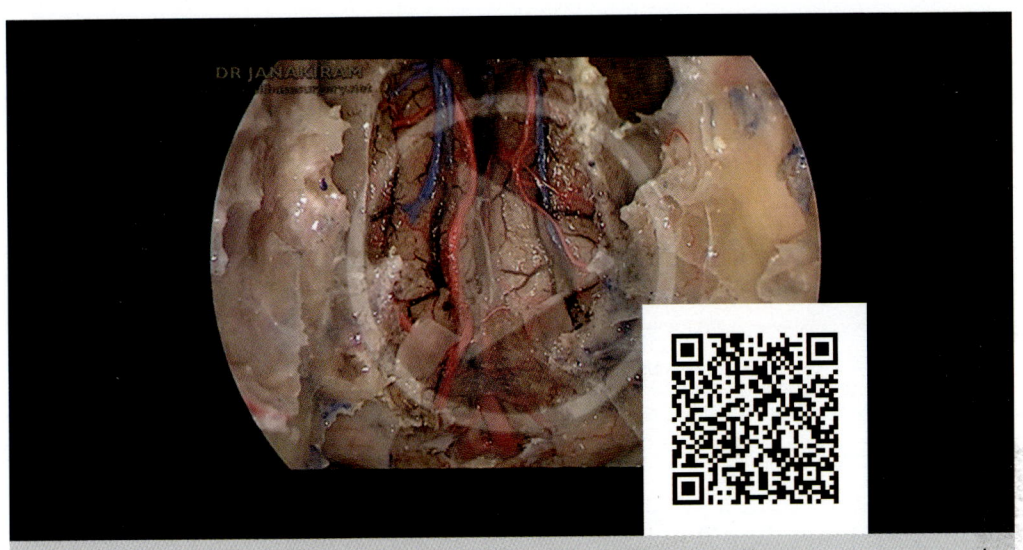

Video 7 Transfrontal approach (DRAF III) and endoscopic transnasal craniectomy approach (ACFR). https://www.thieme.de/de/q.htm?p=opn/tp/388257077/9789388257060_c001_v007&t=video

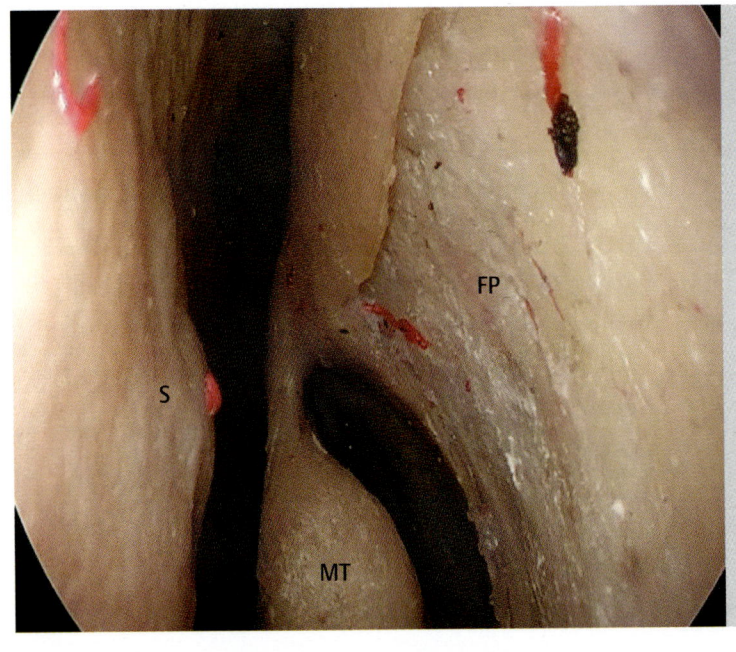

Fig. 7.1 Endoscopic image showing mucosa removed over the frontal process of maxilla (FP) anterior to the axilla of middle turbinate (MT). S, septum.

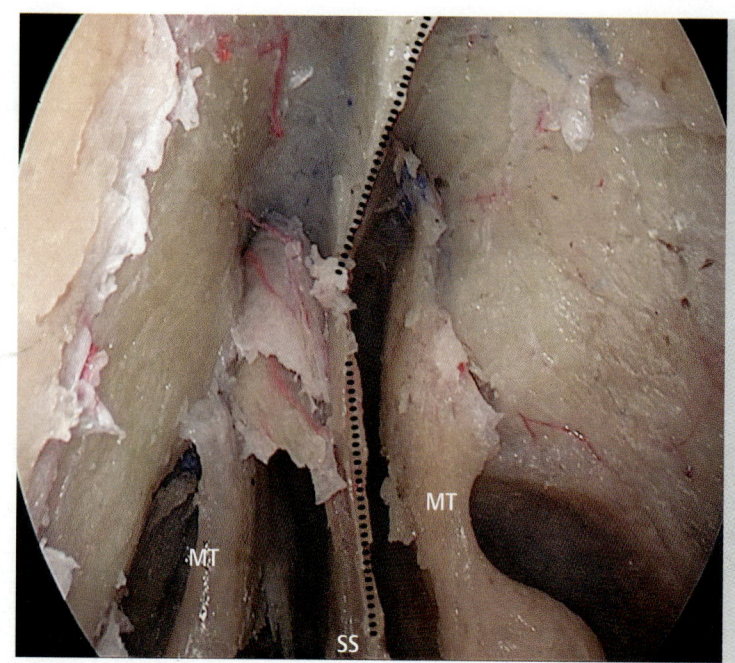

Fig. 7.2 Endoscopic image showing a superior septectomy (SS) in DRAF 3 procedure. MT, middle turbinate.

Now using a sickle knife an inverted U-shaped mucosal incision is taken commencing over the superior part of the septum at the level of the anterior end of the middle turbinate and is carried to the roof and descended over the medial surface of the middle turbinate. The mucoperiosteum is elevated posteriorly along the cribriform area until the first olfactory neuron is visualized superomedially (**Fig. 7.3**). Here the anterior ethmoidal nerve may be initially encountered followed closely by the first olfactory neuron. This marks the posteromedial limit for the out dissection. This structure acts as a landmark to prevent contact with the olfactory groove.

Now shifting to a bi-nostril four-handed approach, the dissector introduces a high-speed drill through the left nostril and suction through the right one. The assistant introduces the endoscope through the right nostril. The drilling (3-mm cutting burr) commences just superior to the lacrimal sac area laterally until a subcutaneous plane is reached and a small area of the skin overlying the lacrimal

Endoscopic Approaches in Sagittal Plane

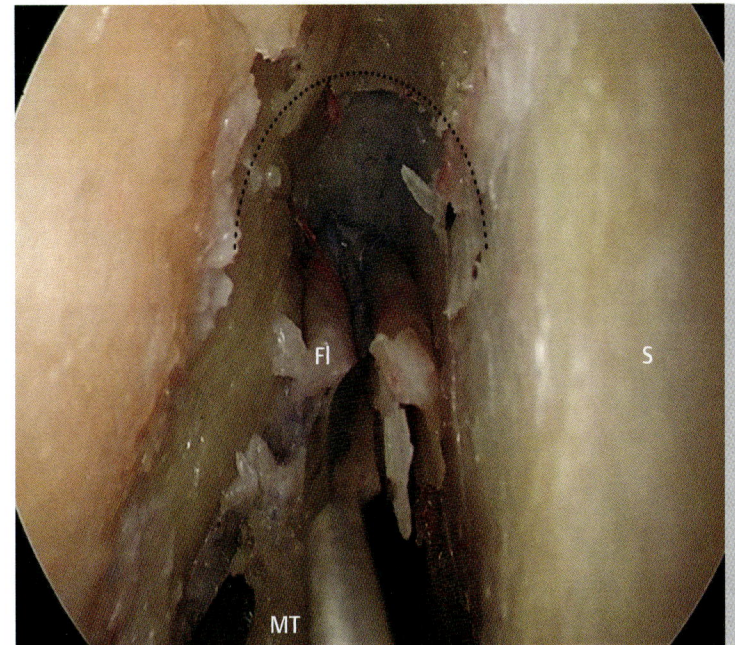

Fig. 7.3 Endoscopic image showing inverted U-shaped incision and subsequent mucoperiosteal flap elevation in the olfactory groove area in U-shaped incision. Fl, flap in the olfactory area; MT, middle turbinate; S, septum.

sac is devoid of any underlying bone (**Fig. 7.4**). This is the anterolateral limit of our dissection. The drilling is continued in superomedial direction. The frontal beak and floor of the frontal sinus is now drilled with a cutting burr. Caution must be exercised at this time to avoid drilling medially. Once the frontal sinus is entered (**Fig. 7.5**) via its inferior wall, the same steps are repeated on the opposite side. Now the openings are drilled medially to combine the two frontal sinuses into a single cavity just above the frontal T (**Fig. 7.6**). The frontal T is formed by the interfrontal septum, perpendicular plate of ethmoid bone, and the superior part of the middle turbinates. The drilling proceeds anterolaterally until the anterior ethmoidal artery is exposed. Now the anterior frontal bone is removed and made flush with the nasal cavity. The intersinus septum is drilled. The forward projecting bone of the skull base at the frontal T is now cautiously drilled (**Fig. 7.7**). The largest possible opening should be created as scaring, and postoperative stenosis reduces the opening to two-thirds of the operative size has been observed over time.

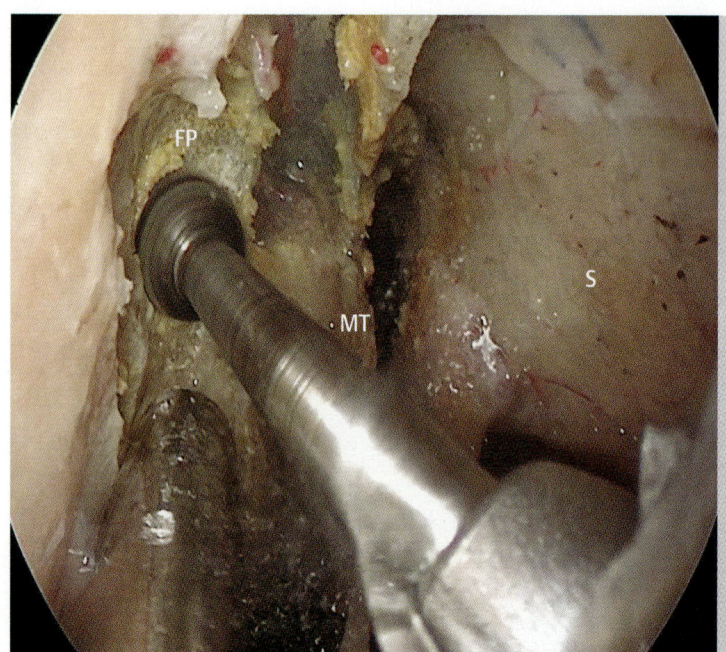

Fig. 7.4 Endoscopic image showing commencement of drilling along the frontal process of maxilla (FP) anterosuperior to the axilla. MT, middle turbinate; S, septum.

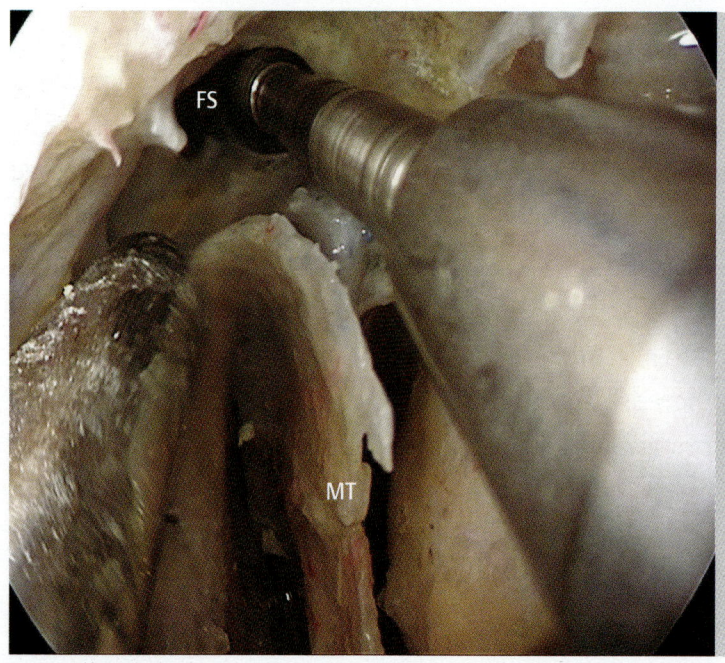

Fig. 7.5 Endoscopic image showing initial entry into the frontal sinus (FS) at its inferior wall. MT, middle turbinate.

Endoscopic Approaches in Sagittal Plane

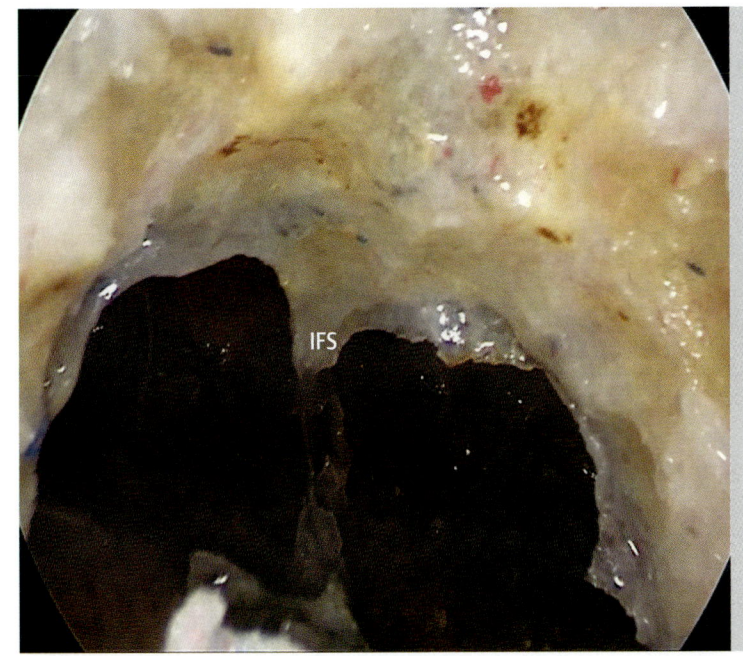

Fig. 7.6 Endoscopic image showing drilling of interfrontal septum (IFS) connecting frontal sinuses on both sides.

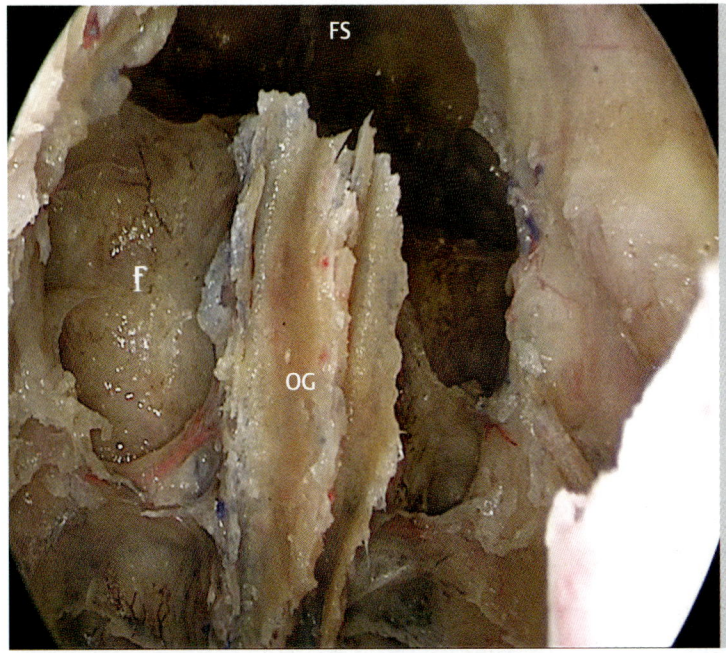

Fig. 7.7 Endoscopic image showing frontal T and the completed DRAF cavity. F, fovea; OG, olfactory groove; FS, frontal sinus.

Reconstruction generally depends on pathology for which the approach is used. CSF leak repairs and tumors with intraoperative CSF leaks are repaired with multilayered reconstruction involving vascularized pedicled flaps. The Hadad nasoseptal flap or alternatively the pericranial flaps are used in these cases. An anterior ethmoidal flap may also be used in these cases to minimize cicatricial stenosis.

Endoscopic Transnasal Craniectomy Approach

The endoscopic transnasal craniectomy approach is implemented primarily for esthesioneuroblastomas and olfactory groove meningiomas; however, midline sinonasal tumors and encephaloceles can also be accessed by this approach. This approach is a transnasal endoscopic anterior craniofacial resection (ACFR).

This approach involves removal of all the structures of the skull base, including the mucosa, sinuses, bone, and dura that is involved by the tumor. The extent of tissue removal depends on the relation of the tumor to the crista galli. However, this approach is contraindicated if the tumor extends far lateral over the orbital roof or in the lateral part of the frontal sinus.

Dissection (Video 7)

A Draf III procedure is performed, and the anterior limit of the dissection is defined at the frontal T. Bilateral anterior and posterior ethmoidectomies with sphenoidotomies are performed. Resection of the middle turbinates and superior turbinates is done bilaterally. With the microdebrider, the mucoperiosteum over the bony part of the posterior nasal septum is removed. Following the posterior septectomy, the rostrum of the sphenoid is removed by lateral and superior osteotomies. The intersphenoidal septum is removed. Now the dissector should identify and access the anterior and posterior ethmoidal arteries on both sides. Cauterizing these arteries in actual cases would devascularize the tumor (**Fig. 7.8**). Now with a high-speed

Endoscopic Approaches in Sagittal Plane

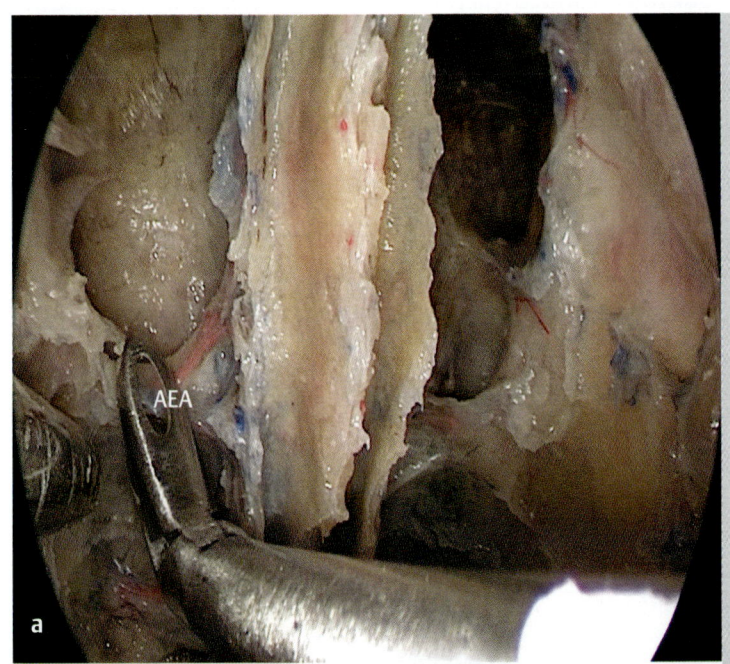

Fig. 7.8 Endoscopic image showing ethmoidal fovea (F). **(a)** Access to anterior ethmoids. **(b)** Access to posterior ethmoids. AEA, anterior ethmoidal artery; PEA, posterior ethmoidal artery.

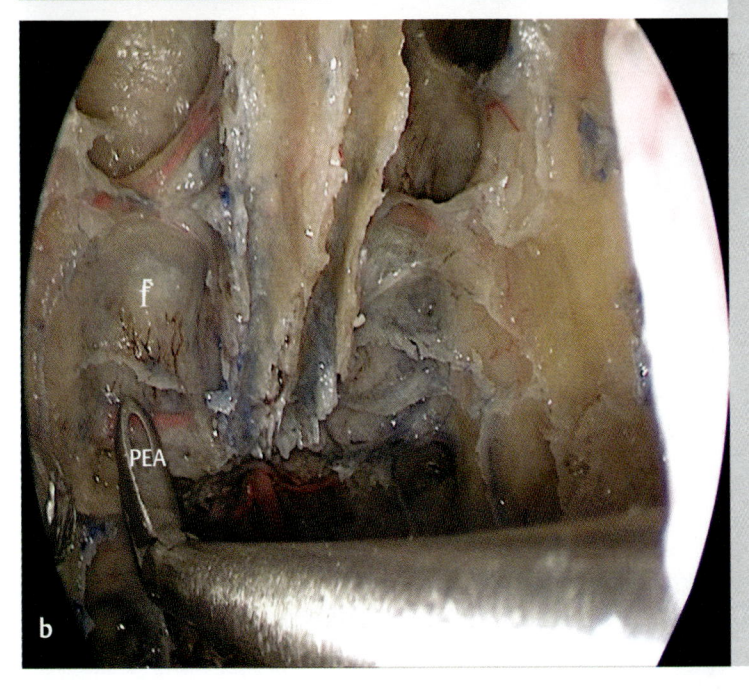

drill adopting the bimanual four-handed technique, the fovea is drilled along its sagittal plane between these two arteries bilaterally (**Fig. 7.9**). The posterior ends of these osteotomies are connected to each other with a planar osteotomy, and an anterior osteotomy above the region of the frontal T is performed. Care should be taken not to injure the dura while drilling. Now the ethmoid roof is attached to the skull base only with the underlying dura. The dura is incised separately with a fine scissors, preferably a skull base Kassam scissors (**Fig. 7.10**). The ethmoid roof with the cribriform plates is now retracted inferiorly (**Fig. 7.11**). At this stage, the falx cerebri is identified and separated with sharp dissection (**Fig. 7.12**). The olfactory tracts are divided with a sharp dissecting scissors bilaterally (**Fig. 7.13**). After removing the ethmoid roof, the frontopolar and the fronto-orbital vessels are visualized (**Fig. 7.14**).

The reconstruction for the large defect created by this approach is done by a pericranial flap. Multilayered reconstruction with allogenic material, fascia, and vascularized flap is recommended.

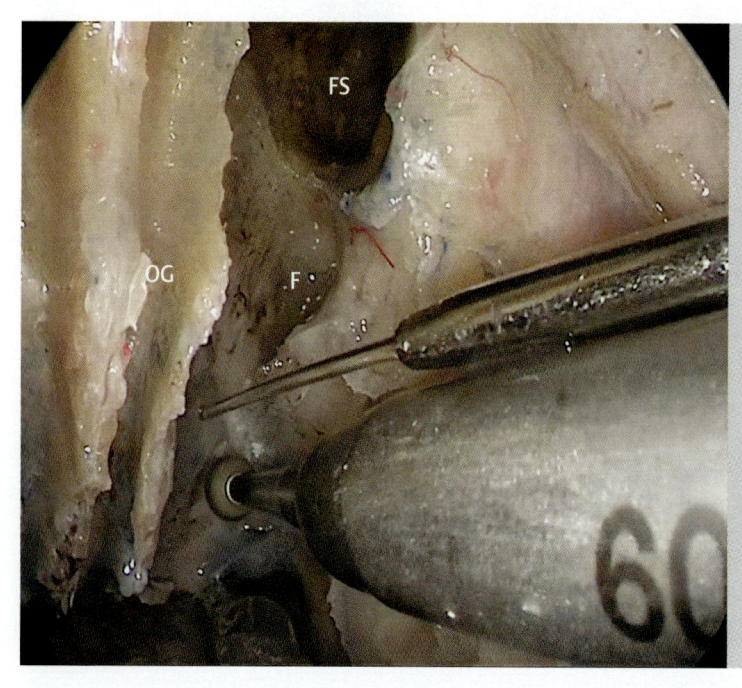

Fig. 7.9 Endoscopic image showing drilling of the fovea (F). FS, frontal sinus; OG, olfactory groove.

Endoscopic Approaches in Sagittal Plane

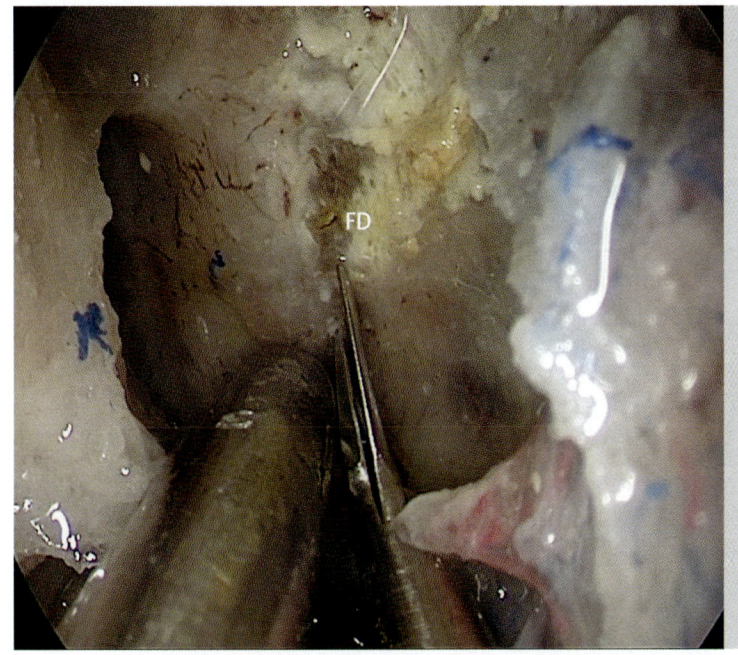

Fig. 7.10 Endoscopic image showing incising of the dura. FD, foveal dura.

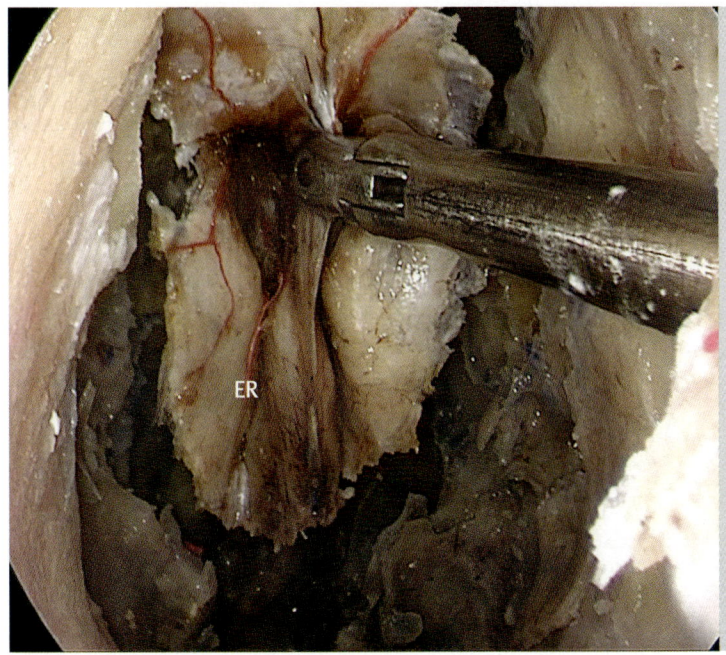

Fig. 7.11 Endoscopic image showing retraction of the ethmoidal roof (ER).

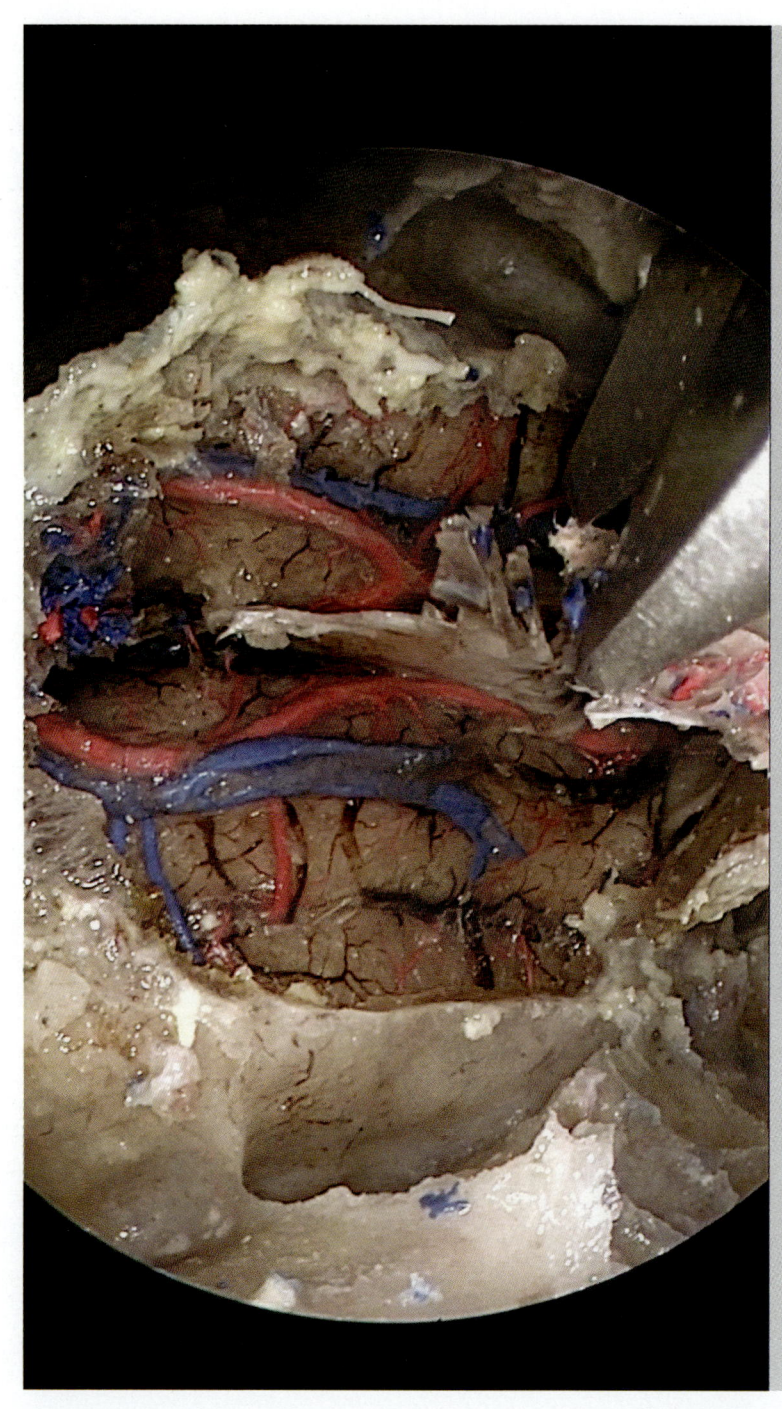

Fig. 7.12 Endoscopic image showing division of falx.

Endoscopic Approaches in Sagittal Plane

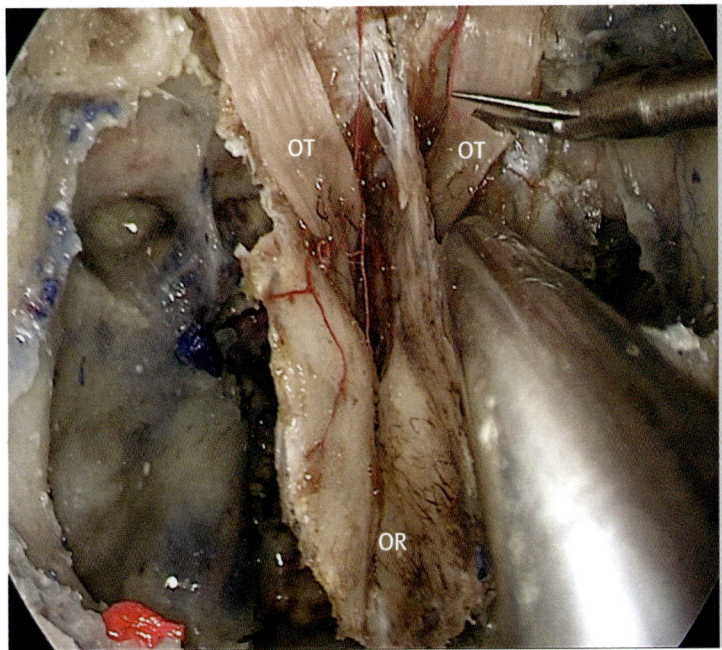

Fig. 7.13 Endoscopic image showing transection of the olfactory tract. OR, olfactory roof; OT, olfactory tract.

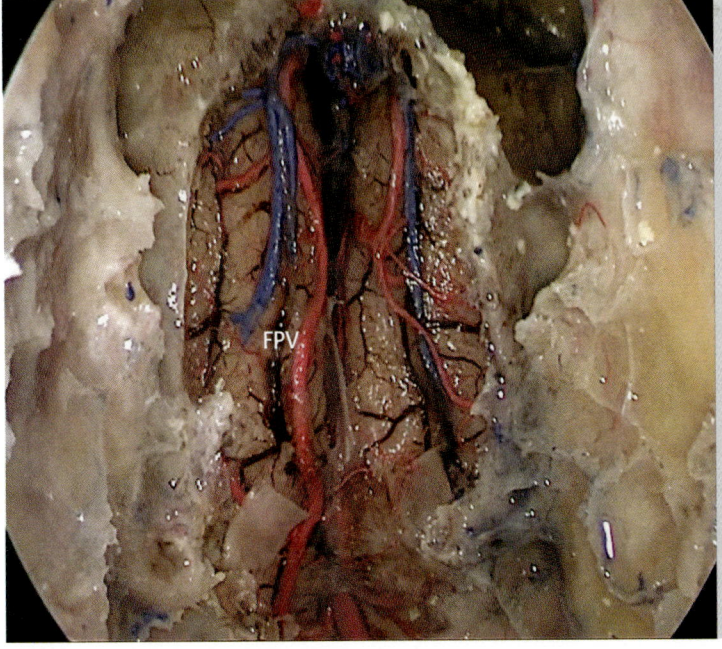

Fig. 7.14 Endoscopic image showing visualization of the frontopolar and frontorbital vessels. FPV, frontopolar vessels.

Chapter 07

Endoscopic Transnasal Transsphenoidal Approaches

Relevant Anatomy (Video 8)

In-depth knowledge of the anatomy of sphenoid sinus is essential for approaching the skull base surgeries. The sphenoid sinus is present as minute cavities within the body of sphenoid during birth. It will reach its full size during adolescent period. Based on degree of pneumatization, the sphenoid sinus is divided into conchal, presellar, and sellar.

- **Conchal type:** The area below the sella is a solid bone without pneumatization and is common in children.

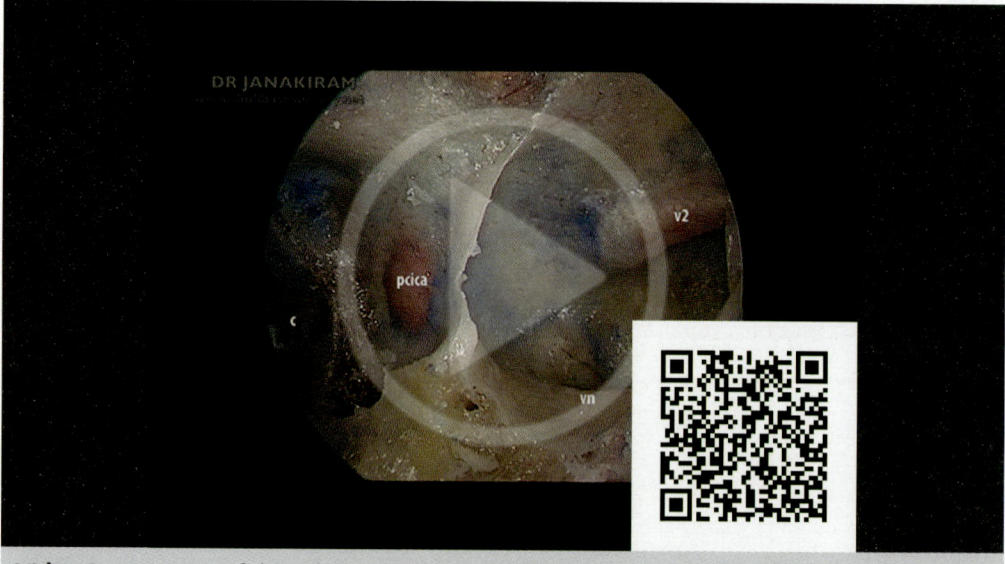

Video 8 Anatomy of the sphenoid. https://www.thieme.de/de/q.htm?p=opn/tp/388257077/9789388257060_c001_v008&t=video

- **Presellar type:** It has moderate air cavity that goes no further than a plane perpendicular to sellar wall (11–24%).[5]
- **Sellar type:** The pneumatization extends into the body of sphenoid below the sella and posteriorly till the clivus and is the most common type.

Extensive pneumatization of sphenoid sinus produces several recesses, which help identify important structures during surgery. The *lateral optic recess* is located between the parasellar internal carotid artery (ICA) and optic nerve along the optic strut of the anterior clinoidal process. The upper and lower edges of this recess mark the upper and lower carotid rings. The part of the ICA that lies between these two rings is called as the clinoidal part of ICA. The *supraoptic recess* that lies above the optic nerve is the pneumatization of anterior ring. *Medial optic carotic recess*, which is the lateral tubercular strut, lies between the medial junction of paraclinoid carotid and optic canal (**Fig. 7.15**). The *lateral recess* extends along the greater

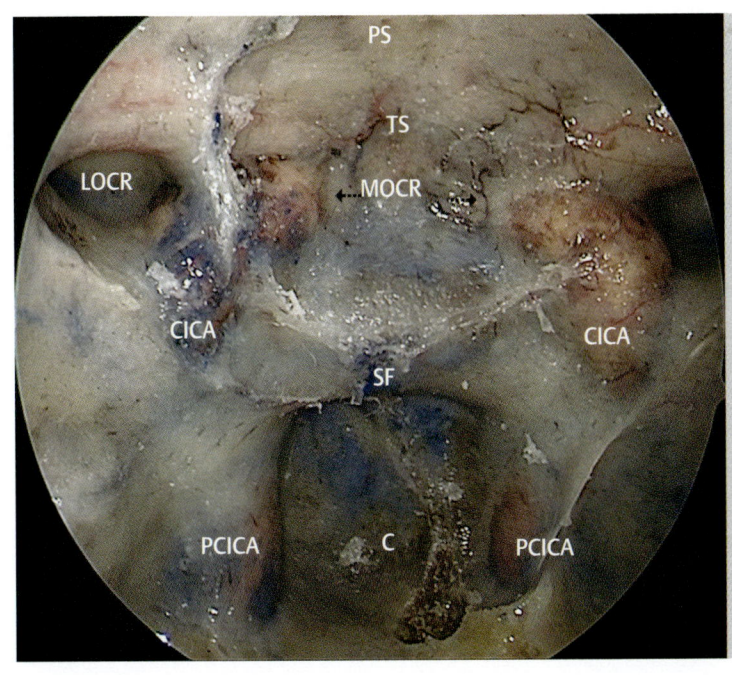

Fig. 7.15 Endoscopic image showing medial and lateral optic carotid recess. C, clivus; CICA, cavernous sinus internal carotid artery; LOCR, lateral optic carotid recess; MOCR, medial optic carotid recess; PCICA, paraclival internal carotid artery; PS, planum sphenoidale; SF, sellar floor; TS, tuberculum sellae.

wing of sphenoid between the maxillary division of trigeminal nerve and lateral to the vidian canal. The sphenoid may extend into the root of pterygoid process called *pterygoid recess*. Anterior extension of sphenoid sinus includes *septal recess*, *superior*, and *inferior ethmoidal recess*.

Sphenoid sinus has an anterior wall, floor, roof, lateral wall, and a posterior wall. The anterior wall of sphenoid sinus contains the sphenoid concha, ostium, a rostrum, and the sphenoidal crest that gets attached to bony septum. An oblique line divides the anterior wall into medial and lateral parts. The lateral part contains sphenoidal concha and posterior ethmoidal cells. The medial part faces the sphenoethmoidal recess. The ostium of the sphenoid sinus opens along the medial part of anterior wall. The trigeminal nerve, optic nerve, and carotid can bulge along the lateral wall, so care is to be taken during surgery (**Fig. 7.16**).

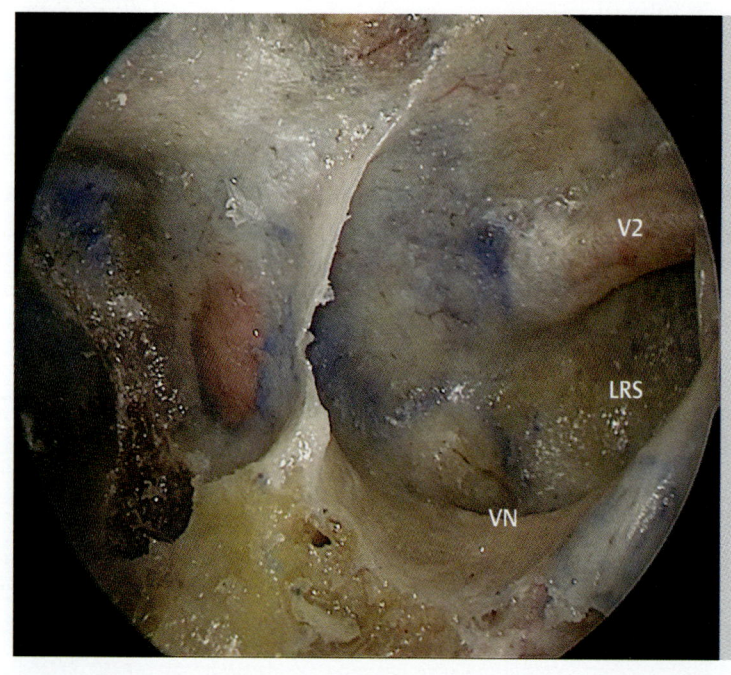

Fig. 7.16 Endoscopic image showing lateral sphenoidal wall. LRS, lateral recess sphenoid; V2, maxillary division of trigeminal nerve; VN, vidian nerve.

The carotid prominence in the sphenoid sinus is divided into three, the retrosellar, infra-, and presellar segments. The *retrosellar segment* is present in the posterolateral part of the sinus. It contains the transition part between the distal petrous and proximal cavernous carotid and is bound laterally by the petrolingual ligament. The distal petrous carotid contains the second or anterior genu, and anterior vertical petrous segment is called *paraclival, lacerum,* or *trigeminal segments*.[6,7] The anterior genu is located above the fibrous cartilage of foramen lacerum. Its lateral aspect lies between lingual process of the sphenoid bone and petrous apex. The anterior genu continues distally with anterior vertical segment and ends in the upper end of petrolingual ligament. Thus, the petrolingual ligament serves as an important landmark for this segment of carotid. The *infrasellar segment* is located below the sellar floor. It contains horizontal part of cavernous carotid. The *presellar segment* is located besides the anterior wall of sphenoid sinus. The cavernous sinus lies on lateral wall of sphenoid sinus extending from infrasellar carotid prominence inferiorly, which corresponds to the superior edge of maxillary division of trigeminal nerve and superiorly up to the optic canal protuberance on superolateral part of the sinus.

The roof of sphenoid extends from the anterior wall of the sinus to the optic canal. It contains planum sphenoidale, prominence of chiasmatic sulcus, and tuberculum sellae. The average distance between the carotid canal in planum is 14 mm.[8] It is possible to approach posteromedial portion of anterior cranial fossa and incisura space, including lamina terminalis and chiasmatic cistern through this corridor. The floor of the sphenoid may be marked by the prominence of the vidian canal. Following the vidian canal posteriorly will end up in the retrosellar carotid.

The posterior wall of the sphenoid can be divided into sellar part superiorly and clival part inferiorly. In the sellar part, pre- and infrasellar carotid prominence marks the lateral limits. On the clival part, the retrosellar carotid prominence marks the lateral limit. The bone over the sellar part is the thinnest around 0.1 to 0.7 mm.[8] Removing the bone over the sellar will expose the sellar dura and intercavernous sinus. This is done during transsphenoidal approach to the sella (**Fig. 7.17**).

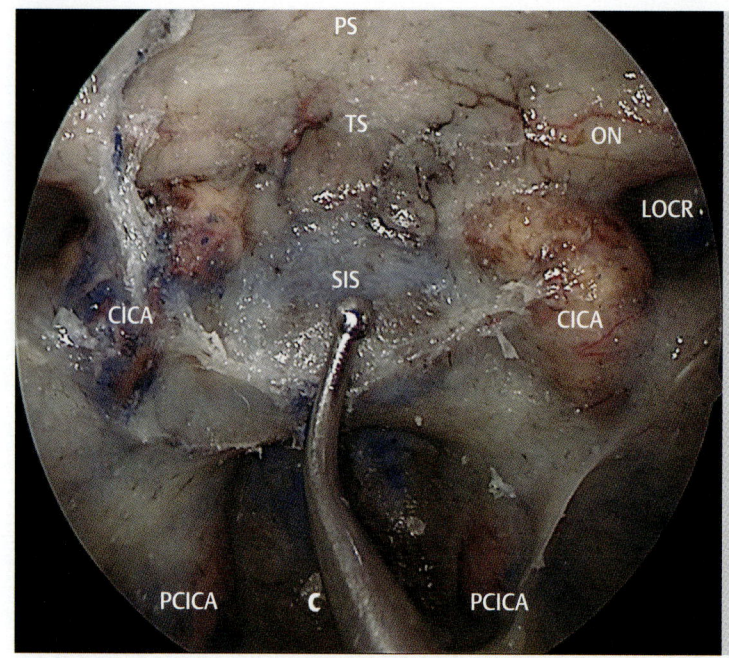

Fig. 7.17 Endoscopic image showing posterior sphenoidal wall. C, clivus; CICA, cavernous sinus internal carotid artery; LOCR, lateral optic carotid recess; ON, optic nerve; PCICA, paraclival internal carotid artery; PS, planum sphenoidal; SIS, superior intercavernous sinus; TS, tuberculum sellae.

Removal of the clival bone exposes the dura of clivus and basilar plexus (**Fig. 7.18**). This area will provide access to the contents of the prepontine and upper part of premedullary cisterns, cerebellomedullary cistern, and medial part of cerebellopontine angle. The sphenoid sinus is supplied by the sphenopalatine artery. The sellar region can also get its blood supply from capsular and inferior hypophyseal artery.

Dissection (Video 9)

The endoscopic endonasal approach to the sagittal planes can be divided into stages such as the nasal phase, sellar, tuberculum, or planar phase. The nasal phase is similar to all approach.

Endoscopic Approaches in Sagittal Plane

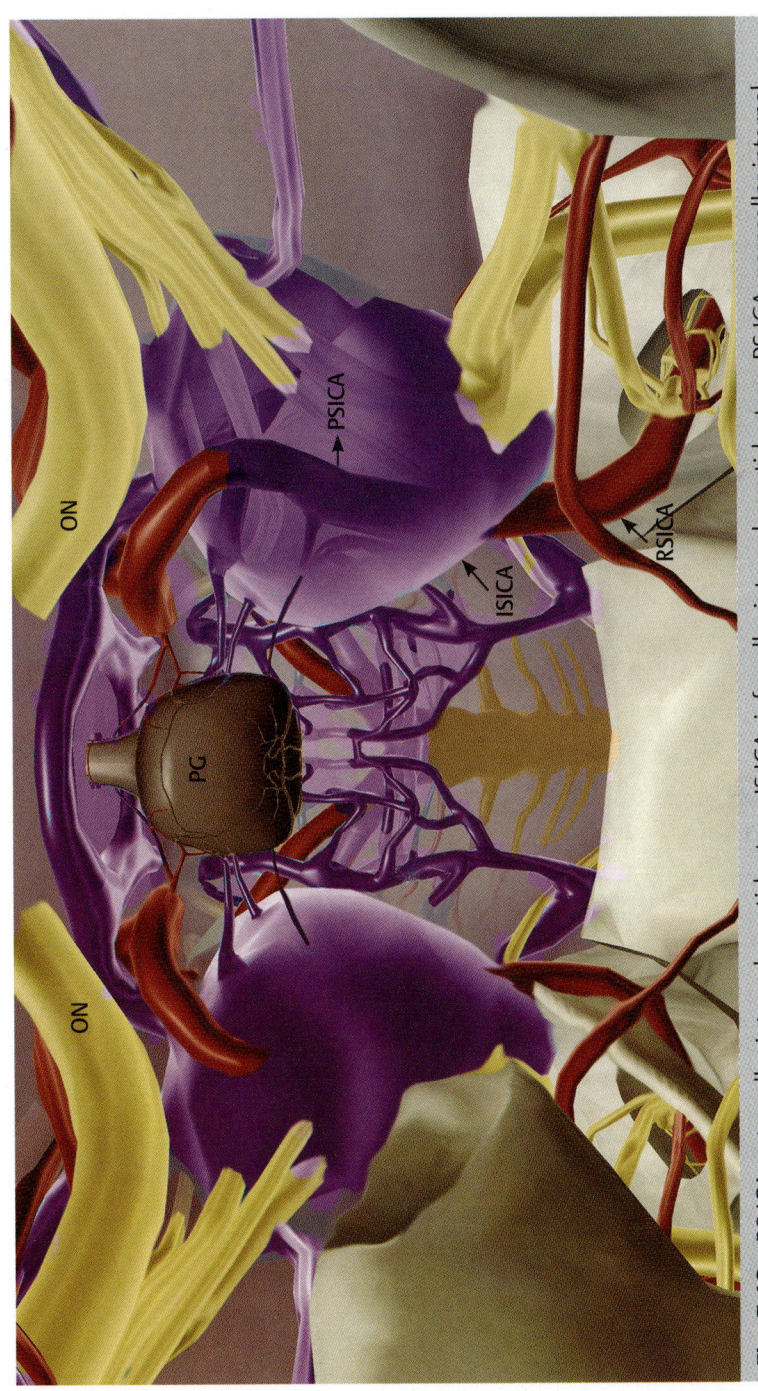

Fig. 7.18 RS ICA, retrosellar internal carotid artery; IS ICA, infrasellar internal carotid artery; PS ICA, parasellar internal carotid artery; PG, pituitary gland; ON, optic nerve.

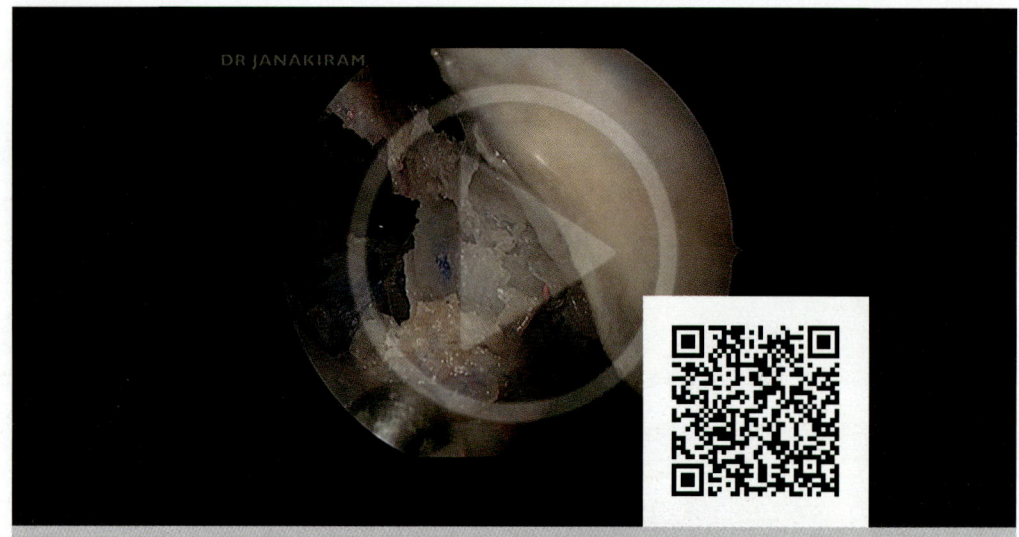

Video 9 Endoscopic transnasal transsphenoidal approach (endoscopic approach to ventral skull base). https://www.thieme.de/de/q.htm?p=opn/tp/388257077/9789388257060_c001_v009&t=video

Nasal Phase

The dissection first starts with lateralization of inferior turbinate on right side with a Freer's elevator. The middle turbinate is identified on the right side, and partial resection of middle turbinate is done (**Fig. 7.19**). Posterior ethmoidectomy is done using debrider. Posterior ethmoidectomy is done to create "a cavity and a half" exposure; the cavity refers to the entire space formed by bilateral sphenoidotomies and the half refers to that formed by posterior ethmoidectomy on one side. This facilitates the dissector to have an unhindered access for instruments. The superior turbinate is visualized, and its inferior part is resected using the through-cut forceps (**Fig. 7.20**). The sphenoid ostium is identified and widened on right side (**Fig. 7.21**). On the left side, inferior and middle turbinates are lateralized, posterior

Endoscopic Approaches in Sagittal Plane

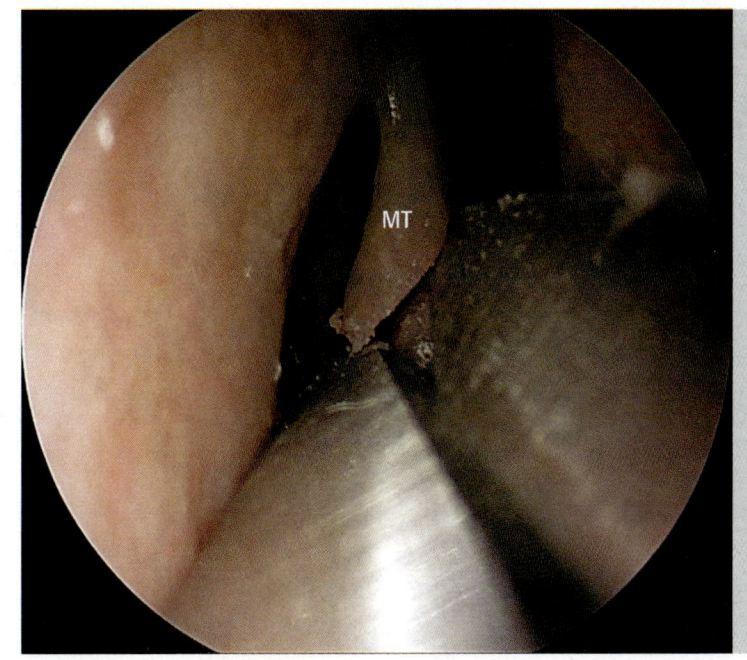

Fig. 7.19 Endoscopic image showing partial resection of middle turbinate (MT).

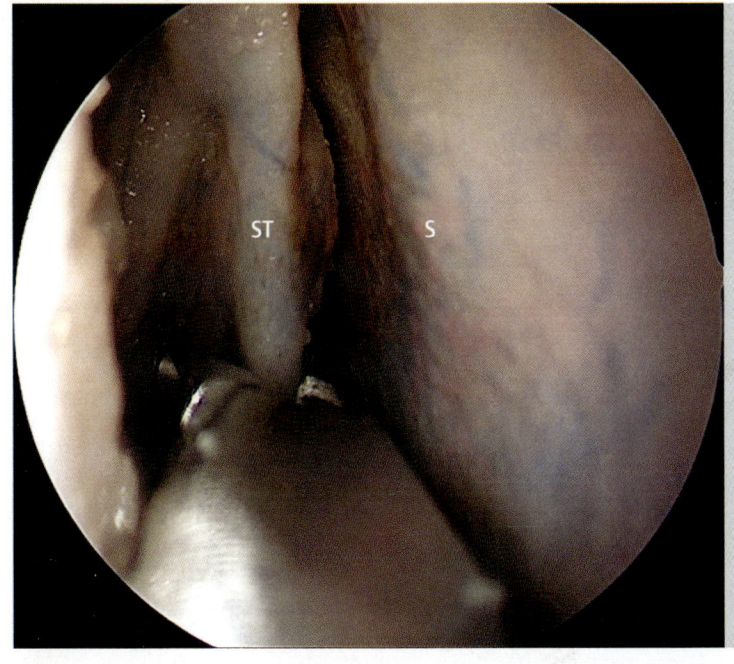

Fig. 7.20 Endoscopic image showing resection of inferior part of superior turbinate (ST). S, septum.

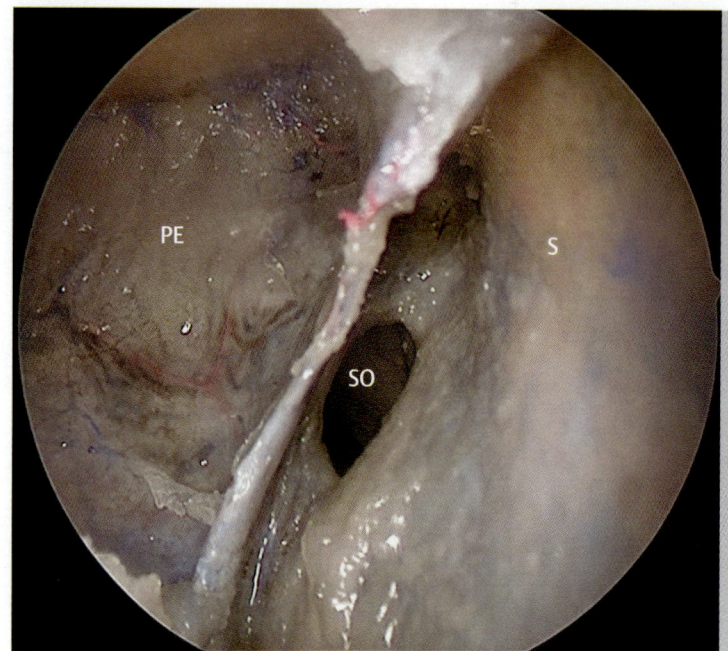

Fig. 7.21 Endoscopic image showing posterior ethmoidectomy and widened sphenoid ostium on one side as a part of the nasal phase in transsphenoidal approach. S, septum; SO, sphenoid os; ST, superior turbinate.

ethmoidectomy is done on left side, superior turbinate on left side is identified, and the lower portion of superior turbinate is resected using through-cut forceps. Sphenoid ostium is identified and widened.

The Hadad flap is raised on the right. Raising of the flap is described in detail in chapter 6 (**Fig. 7.22**). The flap is raised and parked in the nasopharynx. Posterior septectomy is done from the bony cartilaginous junction to the rostrum of sphenoid. The flap on the other side is elevated from the anterior face of sphenoid sinus. The flap on the other side can be taken out as a free flap, rescue flap, or a reverse Hadad flap.

The rostrum of the sphenoid sinus is exposed on both sides fully. Now the four-handed bi-nostril technique is adopted beyond this phase of dissection, and

Endoscopic Approaches in Sagittal Plane

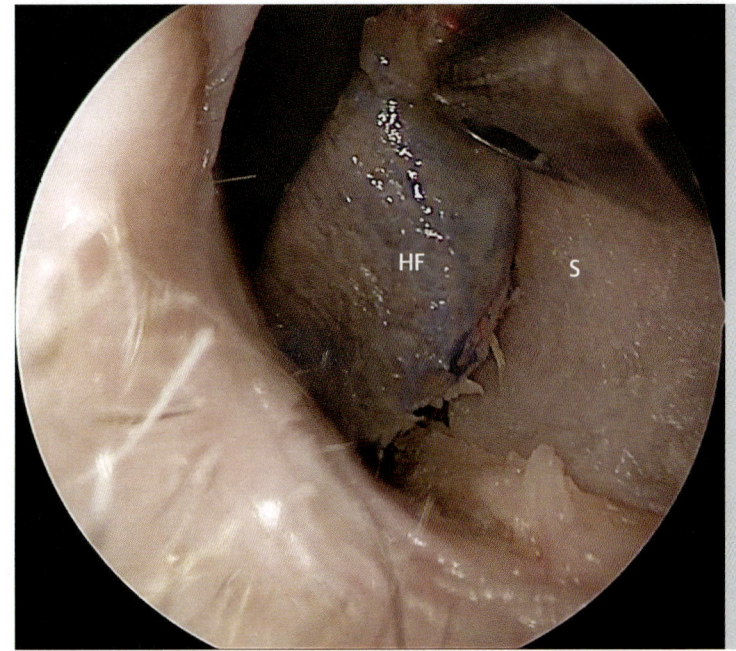

Fig. 7.22 Endoscopic image showing raising of the Hadad flap (HF). S, septum.

an assistant holds the scope and the dissector uses a suction tip in the left hand through the right nostril and instrument in right hand through the left nostril. Karl Storz S III neurodrill with 4-mm diamond burr is used for making osteotomies in the rostrum. First, the planar osteotomy is performed followed by two shoulder osteotomies on the anterior face of sphenoid sinus on either side (**Fig. 7.23**). Care is taken to preserve the pedicle while drilling on the side of the Hadad flap. The two shoulder osteotomies are joined in the floor of the sphenoid sinus. The rostrum of sphenoid sinus is free and can be removed with a Blakesley forceps. The intersphenoidal septum is taken out using 3-mm diamond drill, or with the through-cut forceps, the intersphenoidal septum should never be pulled because it can get attached to the carotid or the optic nerve. The mucosa of sphenoid sinus is removed. This completes the nasal phase of dissection (**Fig. 7.24**).

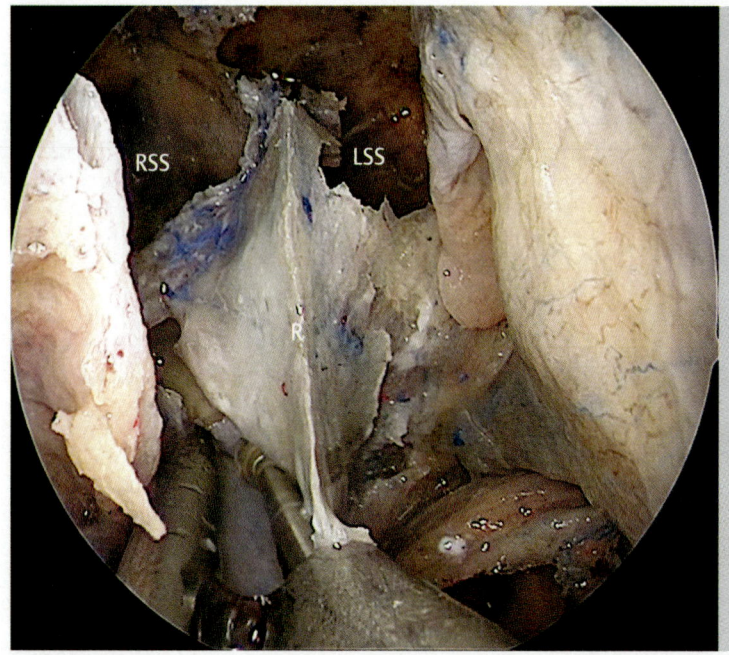

Fig. 7.23 Endoscopic image showing right shoulder osteotomy. Note that in this image planar osteotomy and shoulder osteotomy already performed. LSS, left sphenoid sinus; R, rostrum of sphenoid sinus; RSS, right sphenoid sinus.

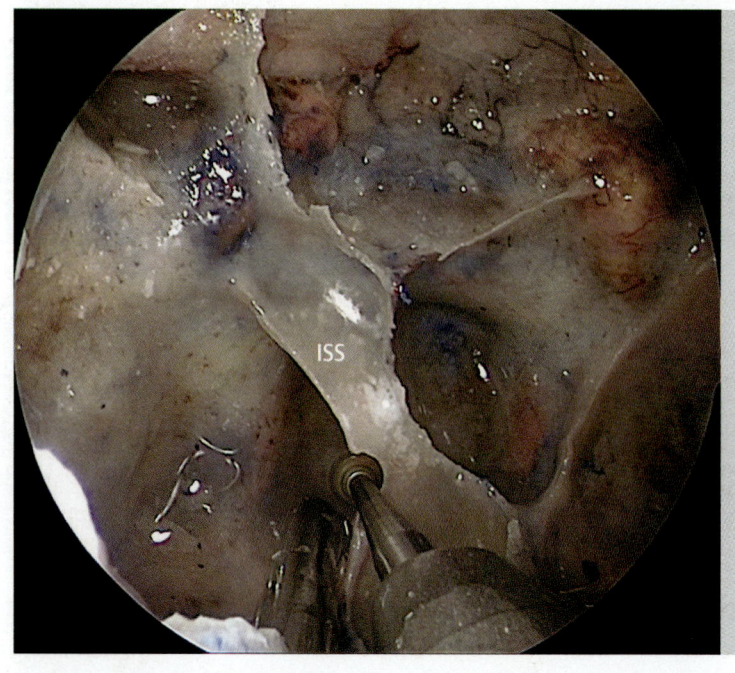

Fig. 7.24 Endoscopic image showing drilling of the intrasphenoidal septum (ISS).

Trans-sellar Approach (Video 10)

This approach is implemented cases of pituitary micro- or macroadenoma occupying the sellar region. The extended approaches such as suprasellar/transplanum are necessary if tumors extend superiorly. Inferior extension of the tumor is accessed by a transclival approach. Dissection in sellar phase begins with the identification of anatomical landmark. The bilateral optic nerve, optic carotid recess, and internal carotid are identified. The sella, planum, tuberculum, and clivus are identified in the midline. The accessory septae in sinus are removed using the 3-mm diamond burr. The floor of sphenoid is drilled up to level of clivus (**Fig. 7.25**). Drilling is done using the 3-mm diamond burr on the sellar face and floor of sella. Drilling is continued until the bone is egg shell thin, and using a Cottle's elevator, the bone over the sellar and floor of sellar is removed. The sellar exposure is

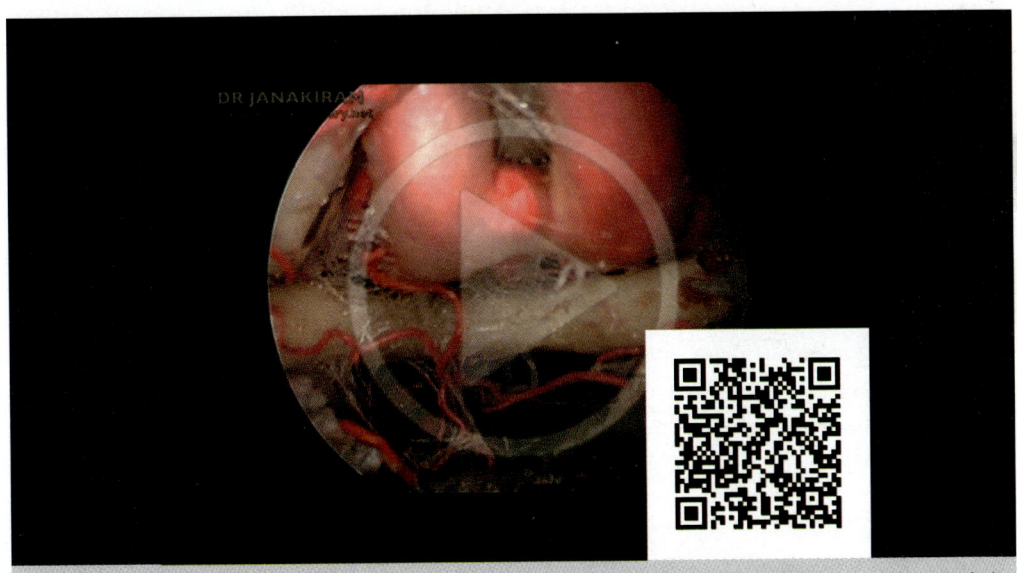

Video 10 Transplanar, trans-sellar, and transtubercular approach. https://www.thieme.de/de/q.htm?p=opn/tp/388257077/9789388257060_c001_v010&t=video

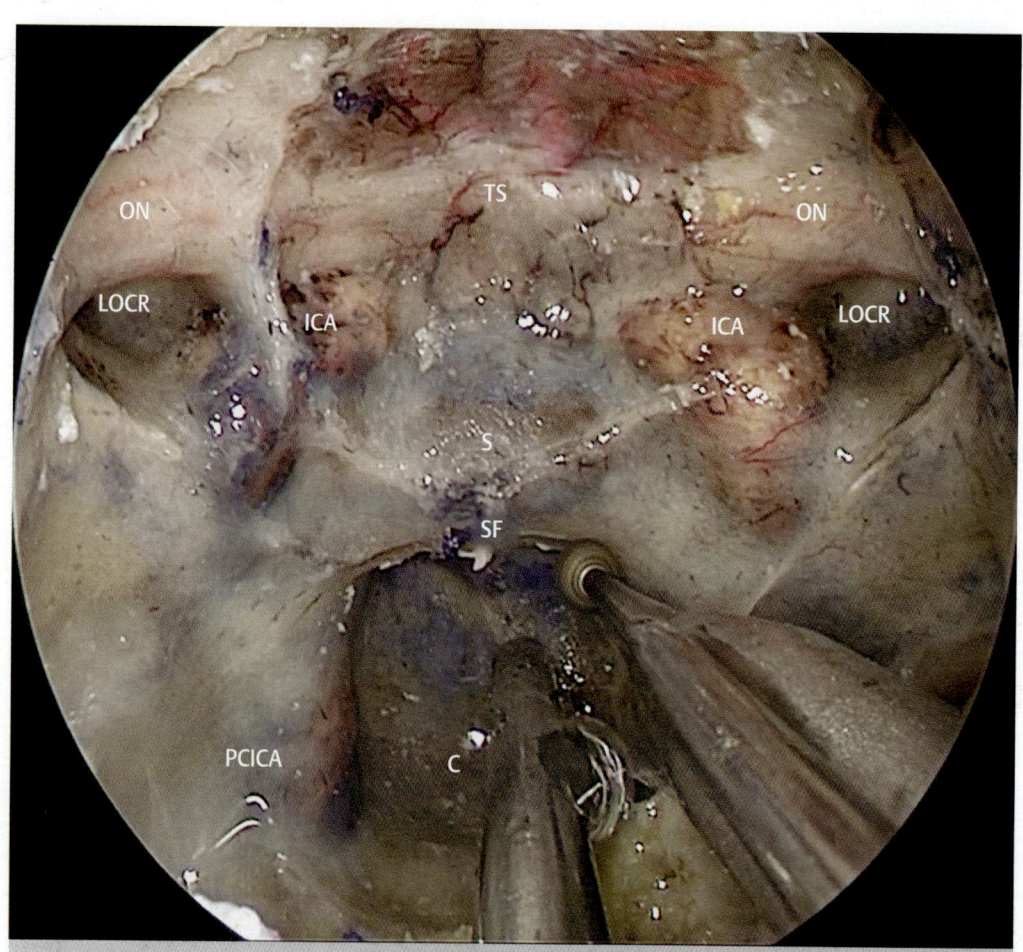

Fig. 7.25 Endoscopic image showing drilling of the sellar bone. C, clivus; CICA, cavernous sinus internal carotid artery; ICA, internal carotid recess; LOCR, lateral optic carotid recess; ON, optic nerve; PCICA, paraclival internal carotid artery; PG, pituitary gland; PICA, paraclival internal carotid artery; S, sellae; SF, sellar floor; TS, tuberculum sellae.

complete with identification of the four blues: the superior intercavernous sinus (SICS) superiorly, inferior intercavernous sinus inferiorly, and cavernous sinuses laterally on either side. The medial-optic carotid recess is drilled on both sides to access the lesion in suprasellar region (**Fig. 7.26**).

The exposed dura has two layers: a meningeal layer that covers the brain and forms diaphragm sellae and endosteal layer that forms the periosteum of the sphenoid bone and extends along the roof and posterolateral wall of cavernous sinus. The incision is made in the dura near the floor of the sella. This incision is taken with Cappabianca knife, and using the Karl Storz dural scissors, a U-shaped flap is elevated. The lateral limit of the flap is the carotid artery, and superiorly it extends till the SICS. Now the pituitary gland with capsule is exposed. With this, the sellar phase of dissection is complete.

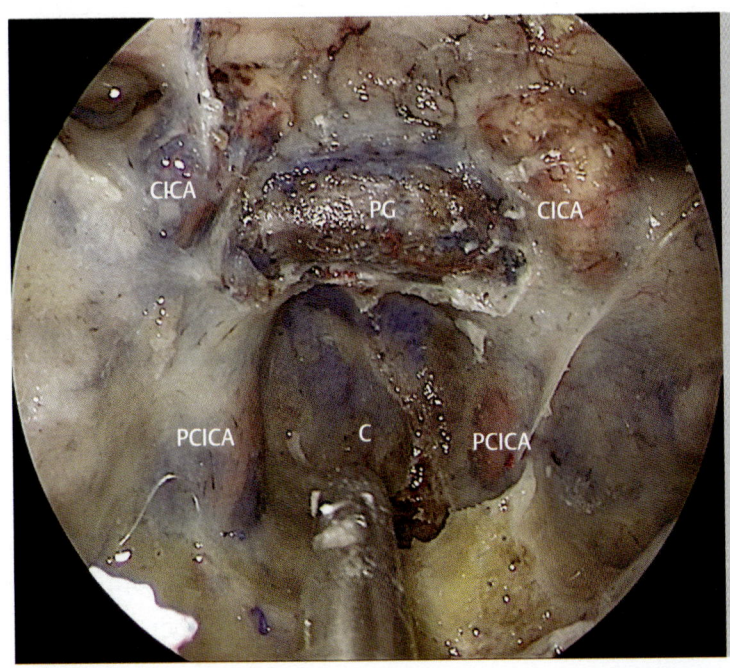

Fig. 7.26 Endoscopic image showing the four blues after complete removal of sellar bone showing cavernous sinus on both sides connected by superior intercavernous and inferior intercavernous. C, clivus; CICA, cavernous sinus internal carotid artery; PG, pituitary gland; PCICA, paraclival internal carotid artery.

Transtuberculum Approach (Video 10)

The lesions of the suprasellar cistern such as giant pituitary macroadenoma, craniopharyngioma and meningioma of tuberculum/planum, epidermoid, gliomas, and tumors of the pituitary can be accessed by this approach.[9] The nasal phase of dissection is similar to this approach. After identifying anatomical landmarks, the bone over the tuberculum between the medial clinoids is drilled using Karl Storz S III neurodrill with 4-mm diamond burr (**Fig. 7.27**). After the bone is drilled eggshell thin, it is removed using Cottle's elevator (**Fig. 7.28**). Inferior bone removal continues halfway up to sellae. Superiorly the bone removal continues in the planum up to the tumor extent. Two horizontal incisions are made in the dura: one above and other below the SICS using Cappabianca knife. The SICS is then isolated. In live surgery, the SICS can be clipped or cauterized and transected (**Fig. 7.29**). Three corridors can be obtained with this approach. The first in front of optic chiasm, the second prechiasmal approach to the third ventricle, and the third is below the chiasm and above the pituitary gland. If the stalk is in between, it can be gently retracted laterally to access the tumor (**Fig. 7.30**).

Transplanum Approach

This approach is adopted for accessing tumors such as craniopharyngiomas, meningiomas, and adenomas.[10] The nasal phase is similar for this approach. The boundaries of planum are posterior ethmoidal artery anteriorly and optic nerve laterally. The osteotomies are made in planum in a triangular fashion using Karl Storz S III neurodrill with 4-mm diamond burr. First osteotomy is made at the base of the triangle just posterior to posterior ethmoidal artery and the two edges of the osteotomies above optic canal (**Fig. 7.31**). The triangular bone over the planum is then removed using Cottle's elevator (**Fig. 7.32**). If the bone over the tuberculum and

Endoscopic Approaches in Sagittal Plane

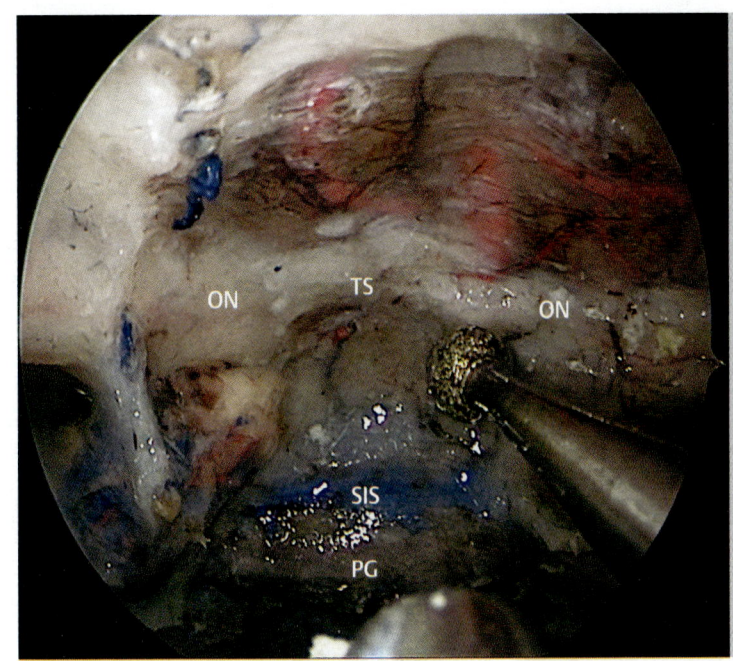

Fig. 7.27 Endoscopic image showing drilling of the tuberculum between the medial clinoids. ON, optic nerve; PG, pituitary gland; SIS, superior intercavernous sinus; TS, tuberculum sellae.

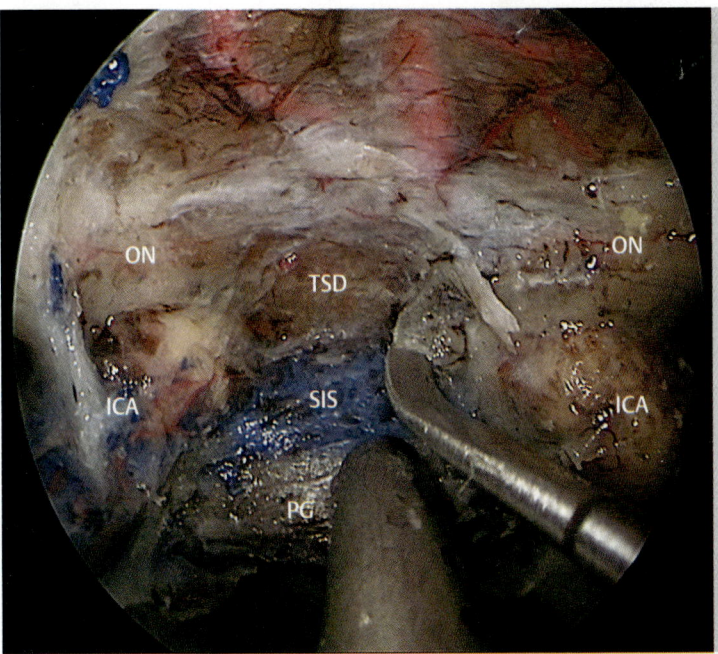

Fig. 7.28 Endoscopic image showing the removal of thin remnant bone over with a Cottle's elevator. ICA, internal carotid artery; ON, optic nerve; PG: pituitary gland; SIS, superior intercavernous sinus; TSD, tuberculum sellae dura.

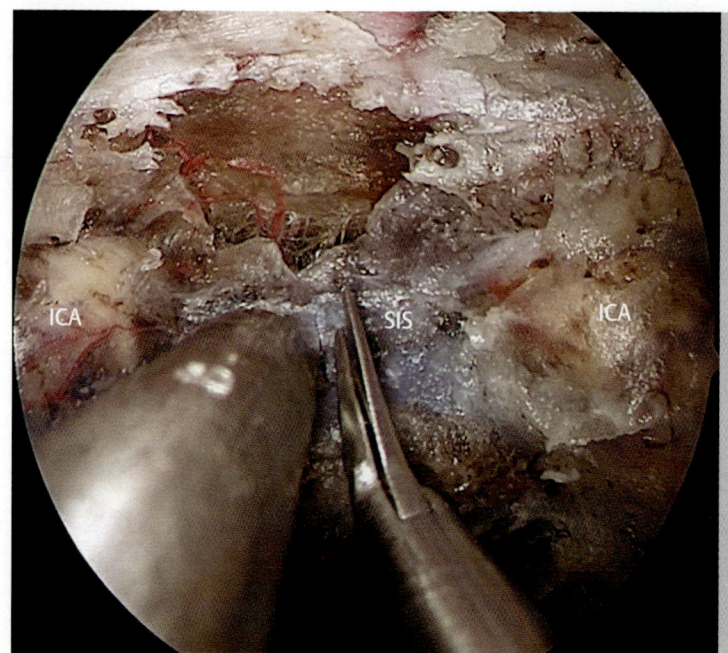

Fig. 7.29 Endoscopic image showing resection of the superior intercavernous sinus (SIS). ICA, internal carotid artery.

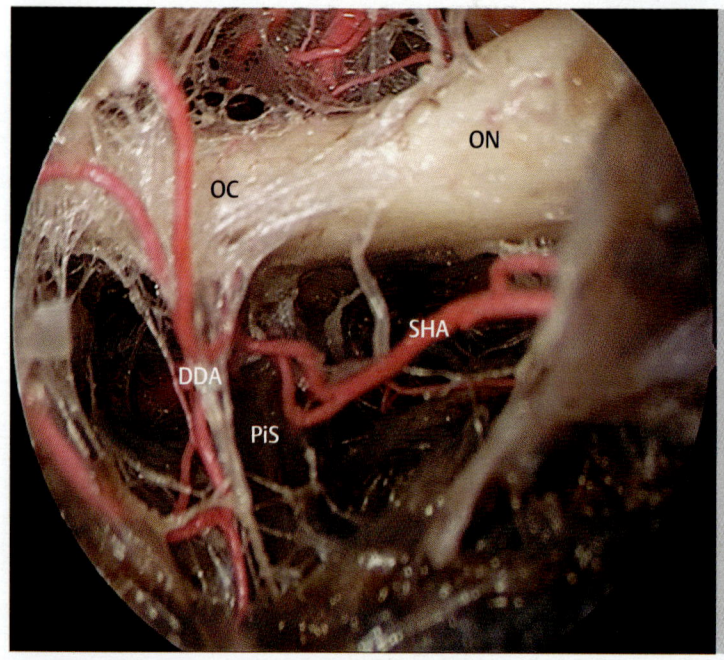

Fig. 7.30 Endoscopic image showing transtubercular trajectories. Note the superior hypophyseal artery (SHA) to the stalk of the pituitary gland. DDA, descending diaphragmatic artery; OC, optic chiasm; ON, optic nerve; PiS, pituitary stalk.

Endoscopic Approaches in Sagittal Plane

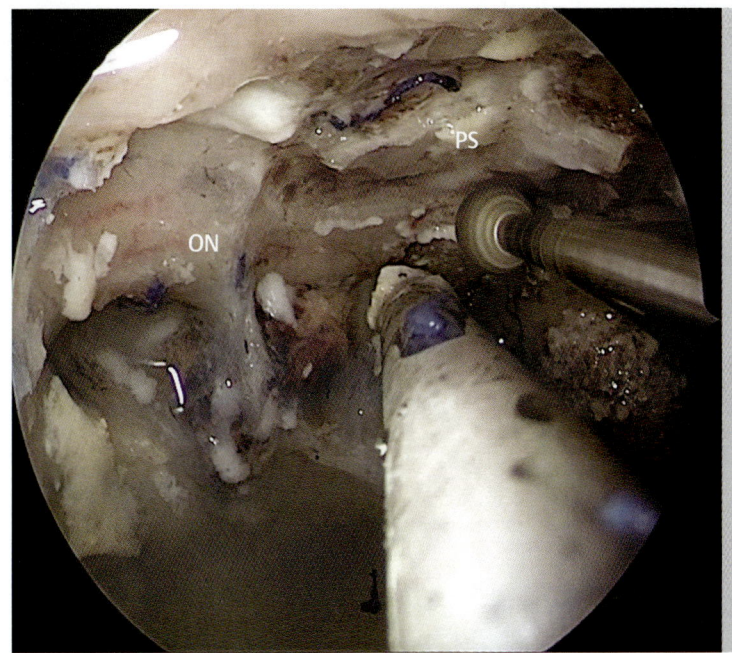

Fig. 7.31 Endoscopic image showing drilling of the sphenoidal planum. ON, optic nerve; PS, planum sphenoidale.

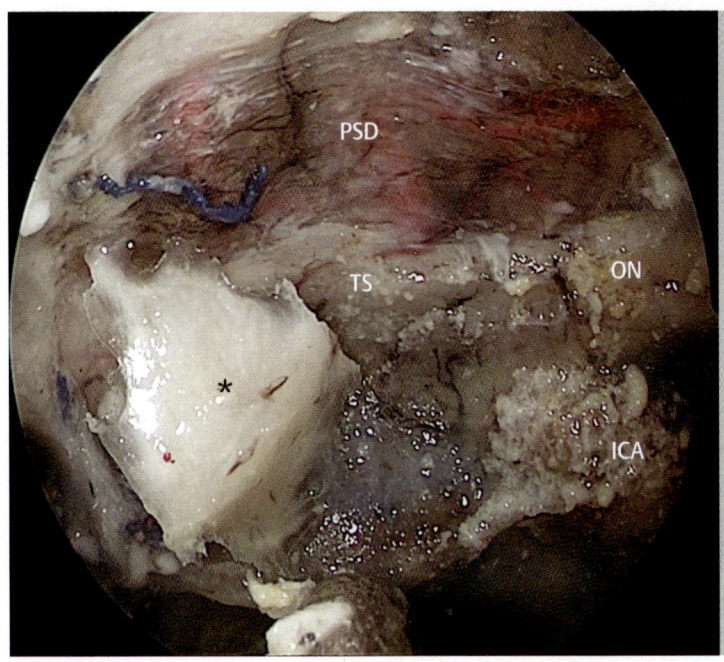

Fig. 7.32 Endoscopic image showing exposure of the planar dura after elevation of the drilled bone. ICA, internal carotid artery; ON, optic nerve; PSD, planum sphenoidale dura; TS, tuberculum sellae.

sella is drilled, this approach constitutes to be a combined trans-sellar transtubercular/transplanar approach. The dura is incised with a Cappabianca knife with two horizontal incisions: one in the frontal dura and one in the sellar dura (**Fig. 7.33**). The vertical incision is made over the SICS joining the two horizontal incisions (in case of live surgery the SICS is clipped or coagulated before making the vertical incision), and the dura is retracted laterally. The optic nerve and optic chiasm are seen in the upper portion, the pituitary stalk is seen in the midline, and either side of the ICA can be visualized.

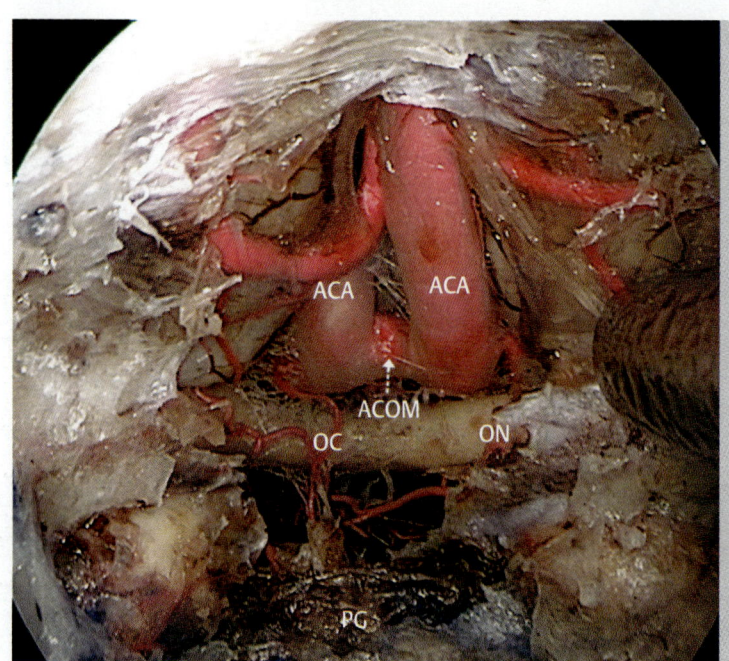

Fig. 7.33 Endoscopic image showing anterior circulation following the resection of the planar dura. ACA, anterior cerebral artery; ACOM, anterior communicating artery; OC, optic chiasm; ON, optic nerve; PG, pituitary gland.

Endoscopic Approaches in Sagittal Plane

Transclival Approach (Videos 11 and 12)

The endoscopic endonasal approach provides access to the entire skull base from the frontal sinus to the craniovertebral junction. In-depth knowledge of anatomy of the clivus and posterior fossa is necessary to access these areas. The clivus is divided into three parts:

- **Upper clivus** extends from the dorsum sellae to the Dorello's canal (canal of the sixth cranial nerve [CN VI]).
- **Mid clivus** is from Dorello's canal till the jugular foramen.
- **Lower clivus** is from the jugular foramen till the hypoglossal canal.

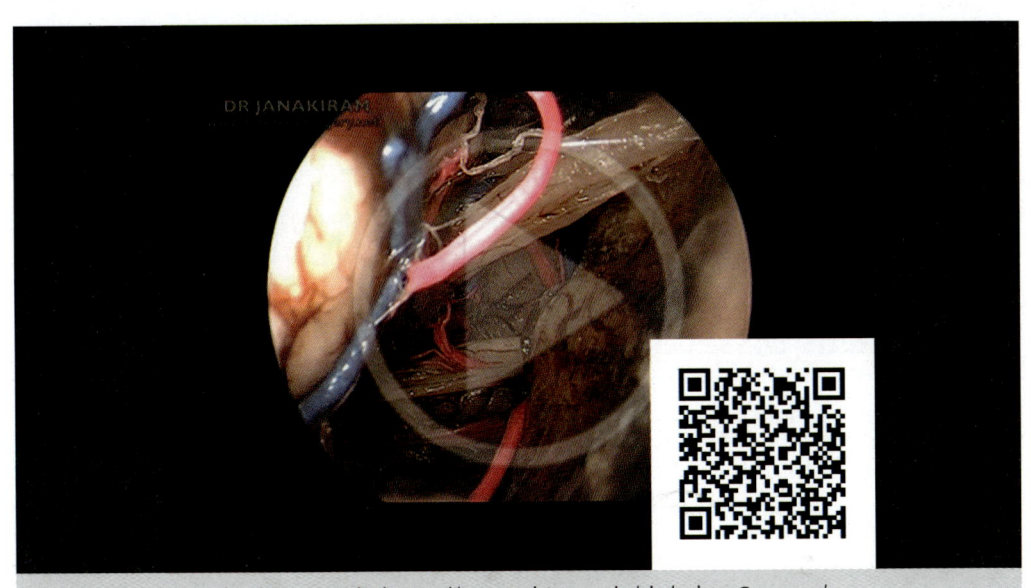

Video 11 Transclival approach. https://www.thieme.de/de/q.htm?p=opn/tp/388257077/9789388257060_c001_v011&t=video

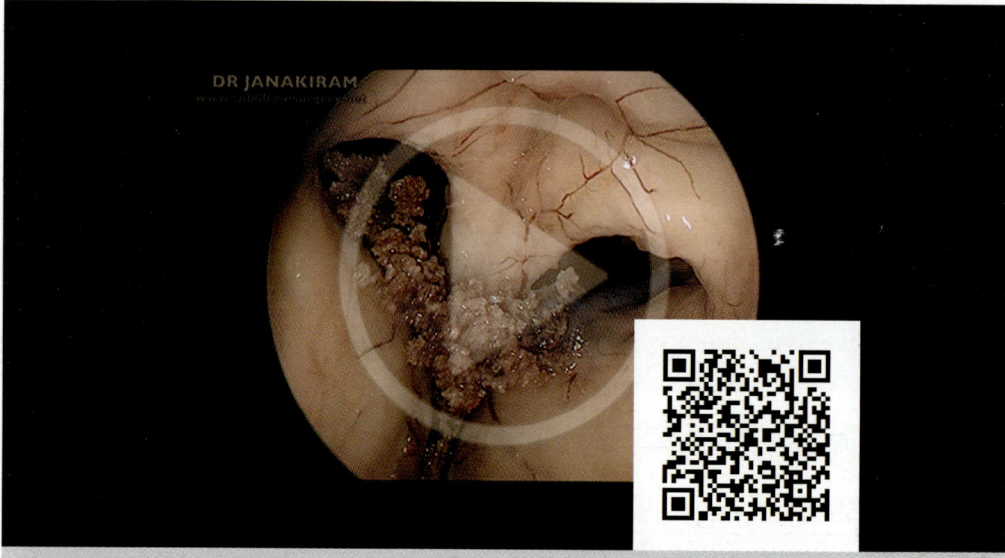

Video 12 Pituitary transposition. https://www.thieme.de/de/q.htm?p=opn/tp/388257077/9789388257060_c001_v012&t=video

The nasal phase of dissection is similar to all transclival approach. The only change is that in the previous approaches, the harvested Hadad flap was placed in the nasopharynx. In transclival approach, a wide middle meatal antrostomy is done on the side of harvested Hadad flap and the flap is then parked in the maxillary sinus.

Upper Clivus Dissection

This approach can be implemented to access tumor occupying the interpeduncular cistern such as craniopharyngiomas, meningiomas, chondromas, chondrosarcomas, teratomas and granular cell tumor, etc. After identification of anatomical landmarks, the four-handed bi-nostril technique is adopted beyond this phase of dissection. The floor of sphenoid is drilled up to level of clivus and the bone over the sella. The tuberculum is drilled egg shell thin, and the bone is removed using the Cottle's elevator. This will expose the dura over the tuberculum and sella. The endosteal layer of the sellar dura is incised near the floor of the sella, and using Karl Storz dural scissors, a U-shaped flap is elevated, the lateral limit being the cavernous sinus. The dura over the SICS is cut, and the dural flap is rotated upward. The pituitary gland is gently elevated with blunt and sharp dissection from the sellar floor as the dissection proceeds laterally (**Fig. 7.34**). The dense dura going toward the cavernous sinus is observed. Elevating the gland laterally will expose the inferior hypophyseal artery branch of meningohypophyseal trunk and numerous ligaments that anchor the pituitary gland. The Pittsburgh group has applied an en bloc transposition technique.[10] This technique emphasizes on complete transposition of the pituitary gland from the fossa, which is achieved by completely cutting the lateral ligaments that anchor the gland to the cavernous sinus. The inferior hypophyseal artery and ligaments are cut (**Fig. 7.35**). The same procedure is done on the other side. Care is taken to preserve the superior hypophyseal artery that serves as the primary blood supply to the pituitary gland. The dura that covers the sella is densely attached to the superior part of the pituitary capsule. After incising that part of the dura, the pituitary gland is free and can be transposed superiorly filling the suprasellar space and prechiasmatic cistern. The live cases gland can be held in its place using the fibrin glue.

This exposes the dorsum sella, which on either side is flanked by the posterior clinoid processes. Two osteotomies are done in a vertical plane along the dorsum sella followed by a horizontal osteotomy in the floor of the dorsum sella (**Fig. 7.36**) connecting the vertical osteotomies. The drilling continues till the dura is exposed. The dura between both posterior clinoid is excised and basilar artery is visualized. The posterior clinoid process on both sides is drilled, thinned and removed using 3mm diamond burr (**Fig. 7.37**). Care is taken not to injure the CN III and carotid artery that are in close proximity to this process. This will expose the interpeduncular cisterns; this cistern contains arteries from the posterior circulation (**Fig. 7.38**). The CN III runs below the posterior cerebellar artery (PCA) and above the superior cerebellar artery (SCA) as it continues to the roof of cavernous sinus. The posterior communicating artery runs posteromedially below the floor of the third ventricle and gives various perforators to the third ventricle (**Fig. 7.39**).

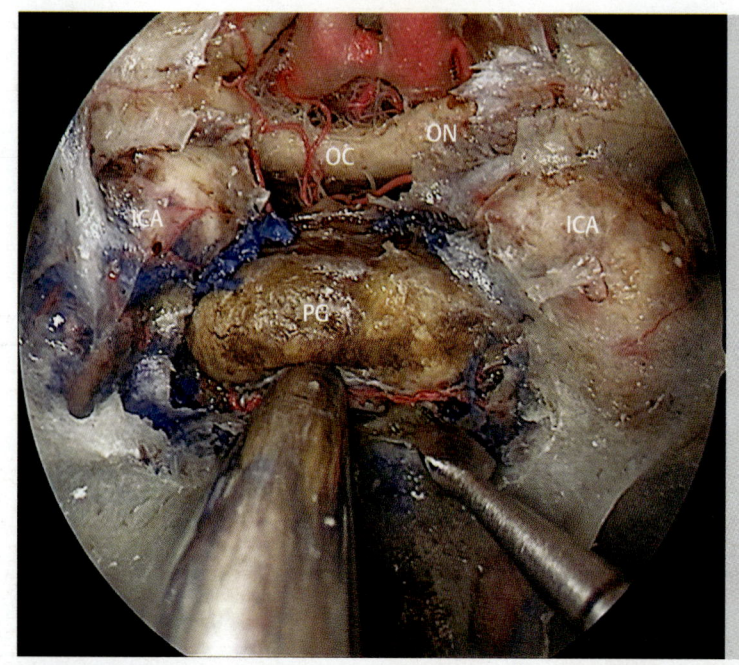

Fig. 7.34 Endoscopic image showing commencement of superior transposition of pituitary gland (PG). ICA, internal carotid artery; OC, optic chiasm; ON, optic nerve.

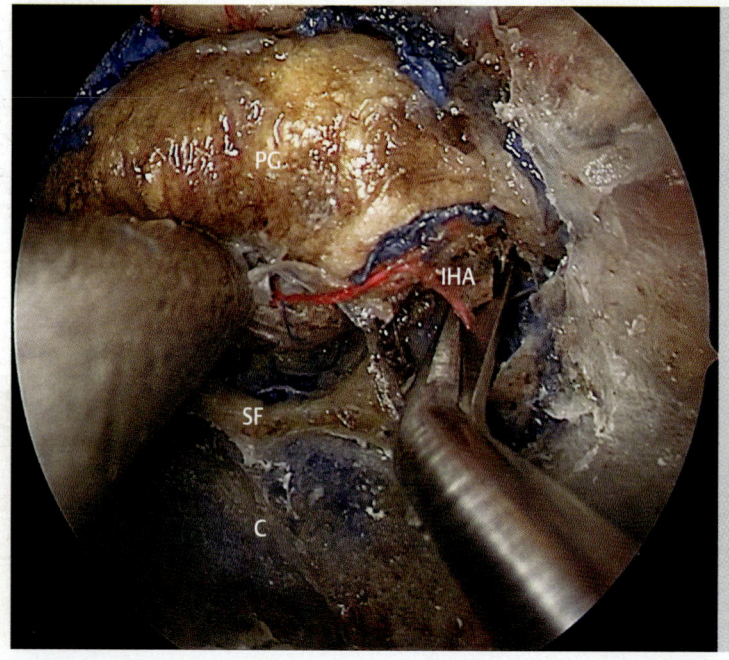

Fig. 7.35 Endoscopic image showing ligation of inferior hypophyseal artery (IHA). C, clivus; PG, pituitary gland; SF, sellar floor.

Endoscopic Approaches in Sagittal Plane

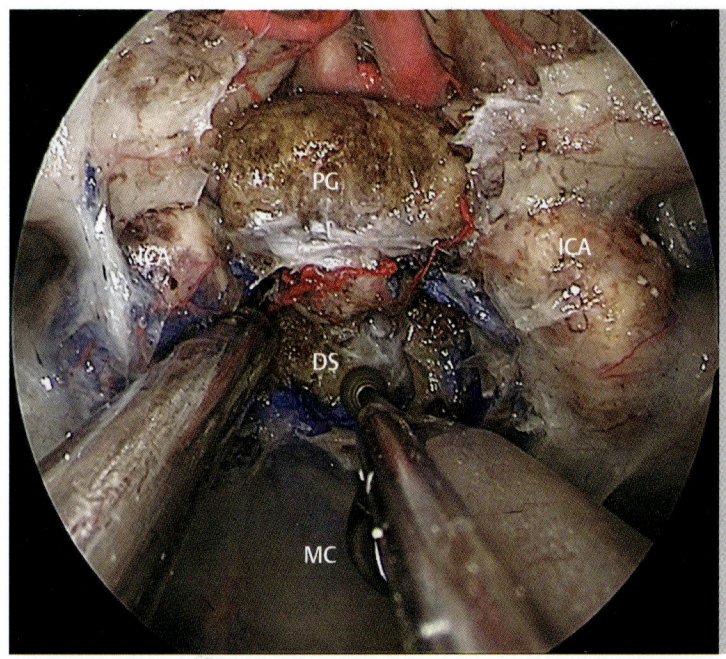

Fig. 7.36 Endoscopic image showing drilling of dorsum sellae (DS). ICA, internal carotid artery; MC, mid clivus; PG, pituitary gland.

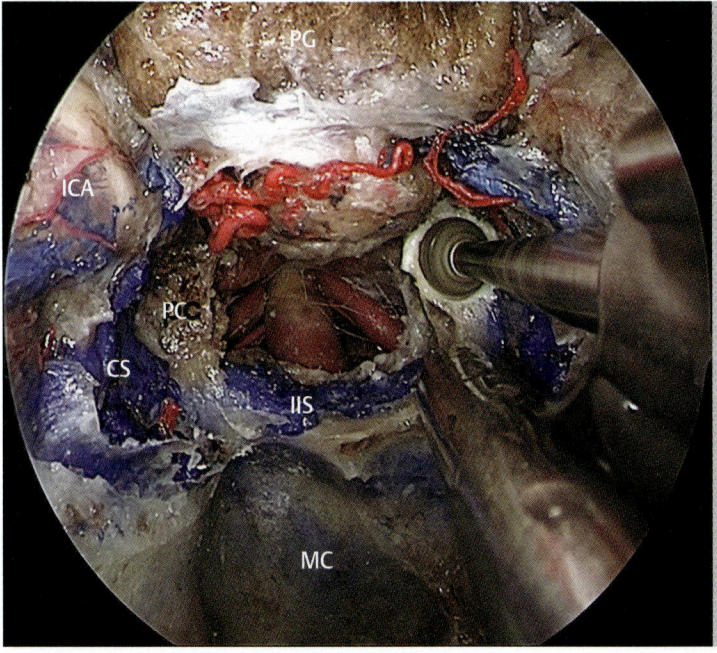

Fig. 7.37 Endoscopic image showing drilling of posterior clinoid (PC). CS, cavernous sinus; ICA, internal carotid artery; IIS, inferior intercavernous sinus; MC, mid clivus; PG, pituitary gland.

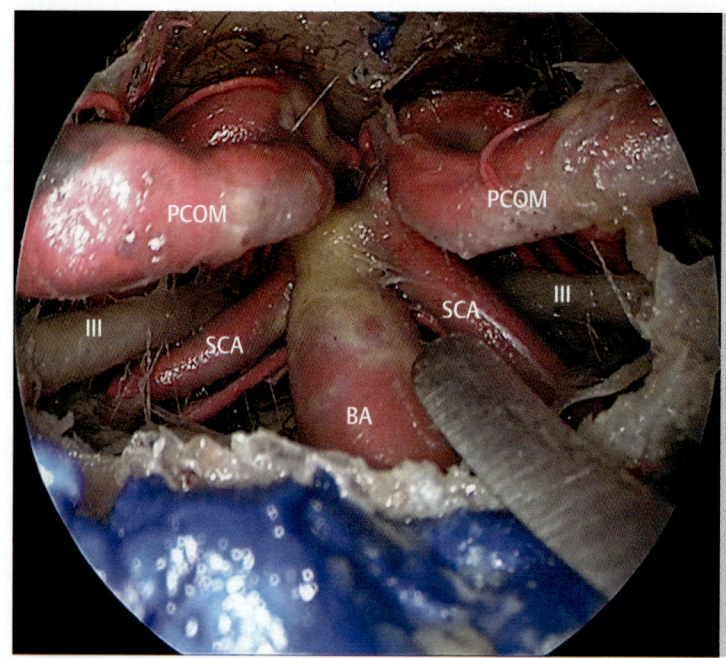

Fig. 7.38 Endoscopic image showing posterior circulation with the oculomotor nerve (III). BA, basilar artery; MB, mamillary bodies; P1, precommunicating segment of posterior cerebellar artery; P2, posterior communicating segment of posterior cerebellar artery; PCOM, posterior communicating artery; SCA, superior cerebellar artery.

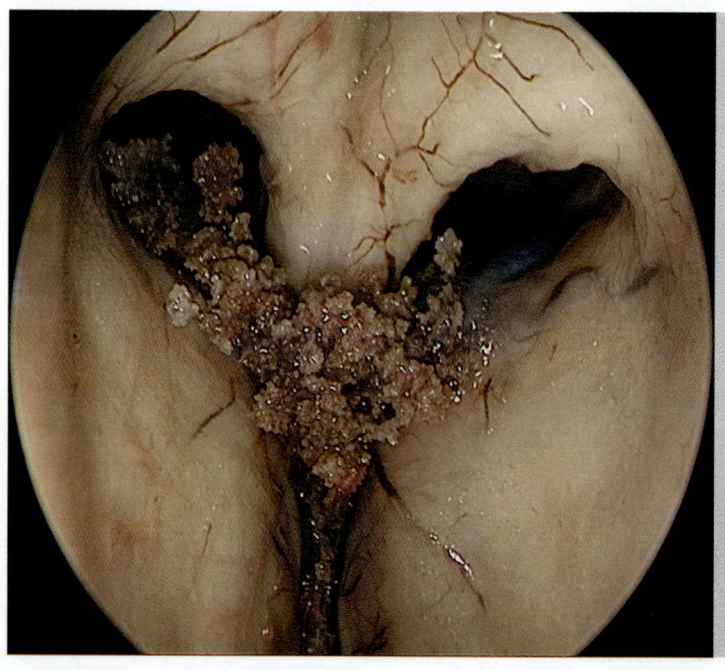

Fig. 7.39 Endoscopic image showing the roof of third ventricle, foramen of Munroe, and choroid plexus.

Mid-clival Dissection

The mid-clival dissection is done for tumors such as meningiomas, chordomas, epidermoid, etc. After identification of anatomical landmarks, the floor of the sphenoid sinus is drilled up to the level of clivus. The mucosa over the mid-clival area is removed. The drilling is done using 3-mm diamond burr from the floor of the sellar to the floor of the sphenoid sinus. Laterally the drilling is limited by the paraclival ICA. The average distance between the paraclival ICAs at this level is around 17 mm.[11] The drilling is continued between these landmarks (**Fig. 7.40**). Here the basilar venous plexus is encountered, which may cause brisk bleeding during live surgery; it can be controlled by Surgicel or FloSeal or by packing with haemostatic agents (**Fig. 7.41**). The CN VI will cross the basilar plexus as it pierces the dura[12] at Dorello's canal that is approximately 20 mm from the posterior clinoid process and approximately 1 cm from the midline. The venous plexus is then cut laterally and excised from the clivus. The dura exposed is cut in T-shaped fashion and retracted laterally. The cisternal segment of the CN VI near the Dorello's canal can be identified. The basilar artery arising from two vertebral arteries can be identified here. The anterior inferior cerebellar artery (AICA) (**Fig. 7.42**) is in inferior relation to the CN VI and the lower cranial nerves lie yet inferior to the AICA (**Fig. 7.43**).

Lower Clivus Dissection

This approach is indicated in case of clival chordomas, chondrosarcomas, cholesterol granulomas, etc. The nasal phase of dissection is similar to that of the upper clivus. Vomer is drilled up to the level of hard palate. The mucosa of the lower clivus is removed using cold steal instruments during dissection, but in surgery a Coblator is used. After the mucosa is excised, the longus capitis and longus colli muscle are exposed (**Fig. 7.44**). The buccopharyngeal fascia is incised, and the muscle is elevated and dissected to expose basisphenoid and basioccipital. Drilling is done using a 3-mm cutting burr. Drilling can extend laterally in this area as the paraclival carotid artery in the mid-clivus continues as petrous carotid artery enclosed

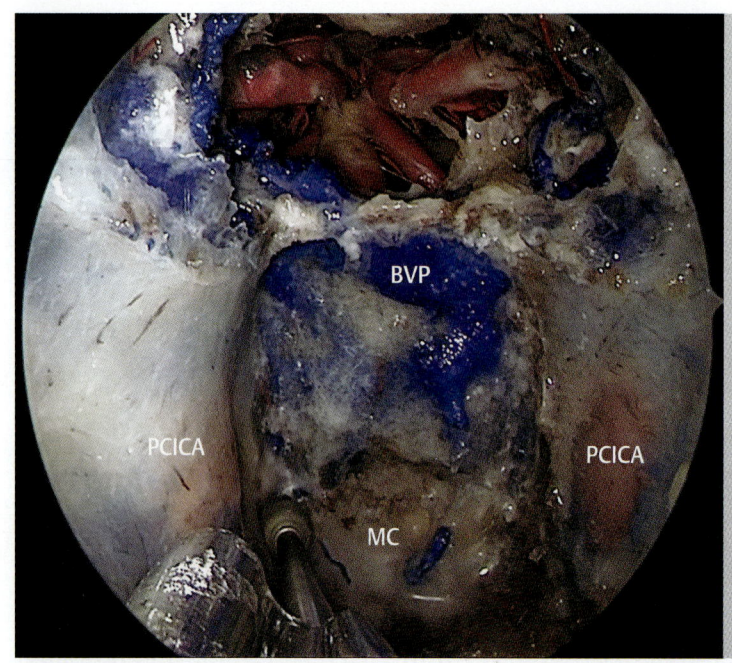

Fig. 7.40 Endoscopic image showing drilling of the mid clivus (MC). BVP, basilar venus plexus; PCICA, paraclival internal carotid artery.

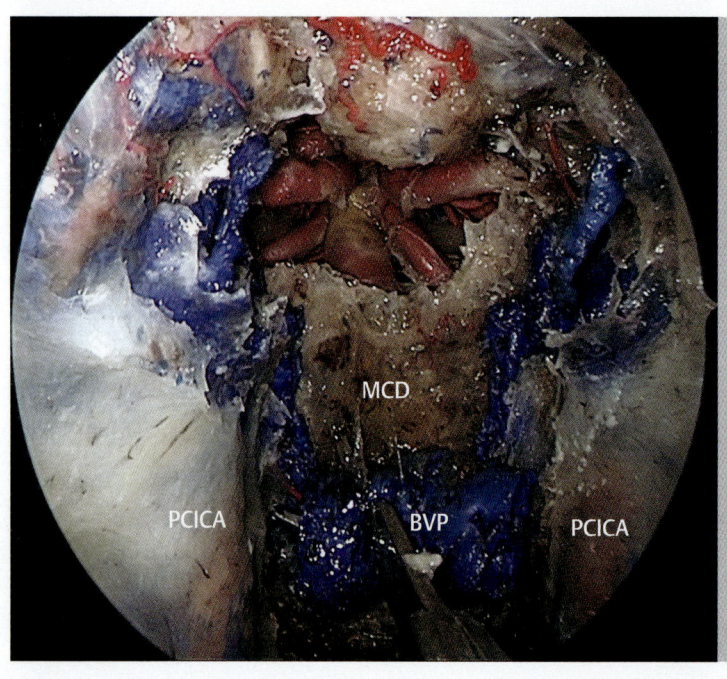

Fig. 7.41 Endoscopic image showing resection of basilar venous plexus (BVP). MCD, mid clival dura; PCICA, paraclival internal carotid artery.

Endoscopic Approaches in Sagittal Plane 149

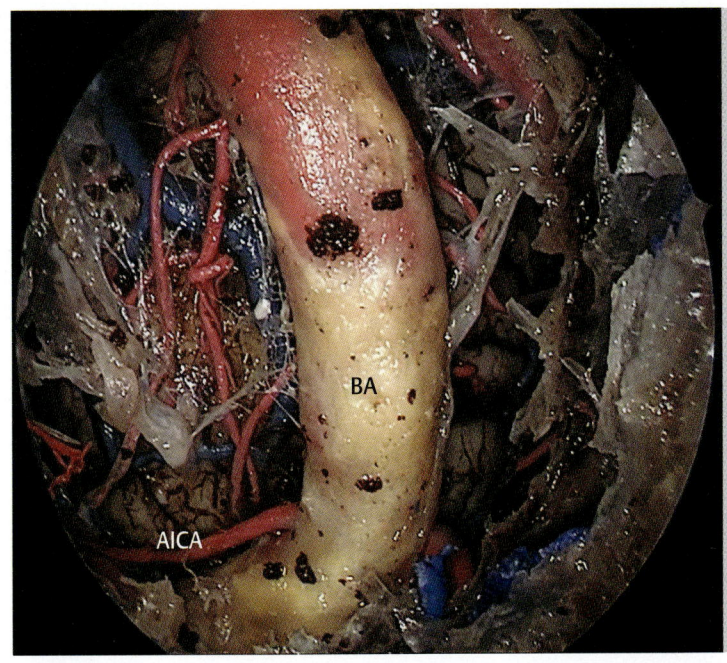

Fig. 7.42 Endoscopic image showing complete exposure of the mid clival and the anterior inferior cerebellar artery (AICA). BA, basilar artery.

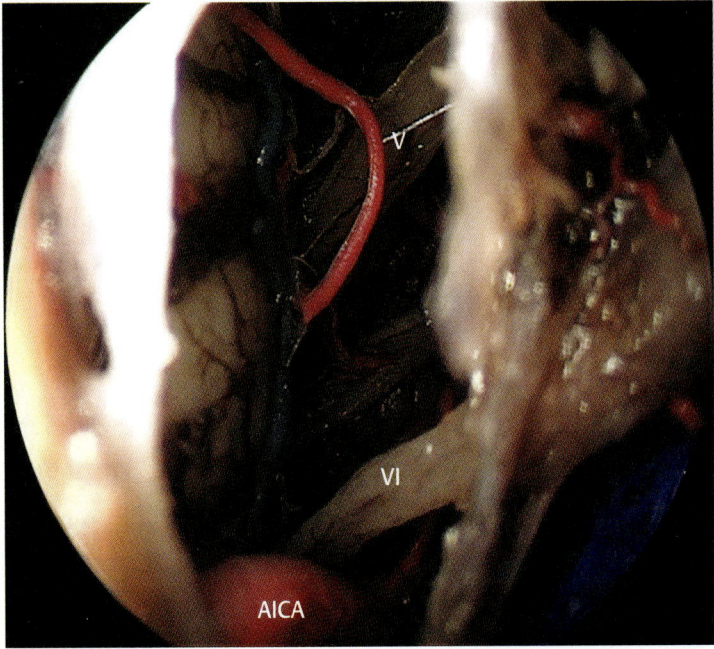

Fig. 7.43 Endoscopic image showing the sixth cranial nerve after complete dissection of mid clivus. AICA, anterior inferior cerebellar; V, trigeminal nerve; VI, abducent nerve.

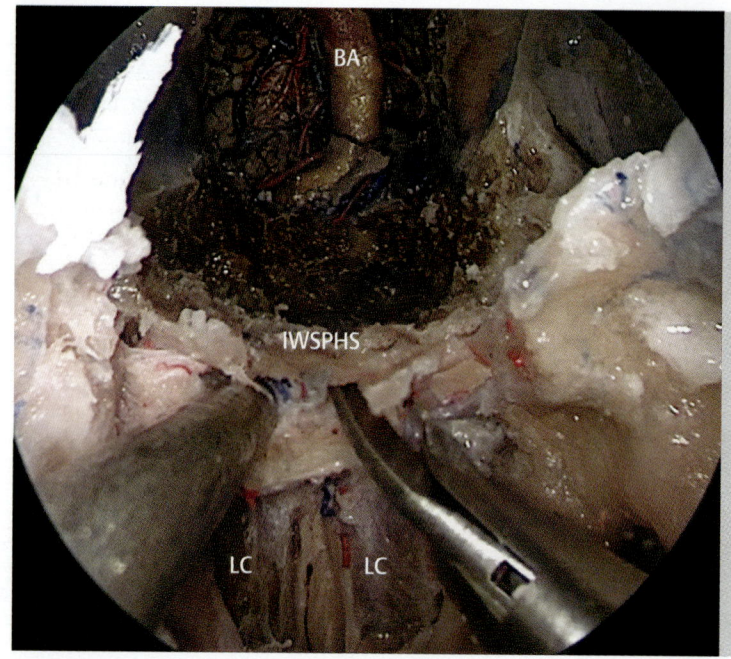

Fig. 7.44 Endoscopic image showing exposure of basisphenoid and basioccipital with resection of longus colli and longus capitis (LC). BA, basilar artery; IWSPHS, inferior wall of sphenoid sinus.

in its bony canal (**Fig. 7.45**). The lower limit of drilling is up to the arch of atlas. The exposed dura is incised in the midline and retracted laterally. The lateral limit of exposure is the hypoglossal canal. The hypoglossal nerve is identified (**Fig. 7.46**). The vertebral artery and origin of the posterior inferior cerebellar artery (PICA) (**Fig. 7.47**), and the anterior spinal vessels are identified. This completes the dissection to the lower clivus.

Reconstruction

Reconstruction[13] options for all these approaches in the sagittal plane depend on the pathology. At the authors' center, a multilayer closure with Hadad flap, lateral nasal wall, or, alternatively, the pericranial flap is adopted, depending on the size of the defect and availability of flap. The multilayer reconstruction is first with fat, which can obliterate the dead space and then with the soft tissue graft fascia lata,

Endoscopic Approaches in Sagittal Plane

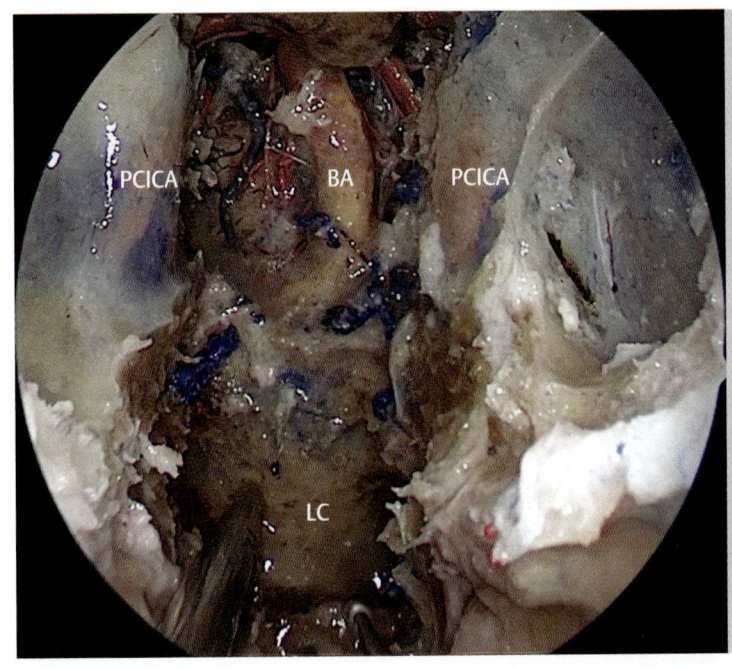

Fig. 7.45 Endoscopic image showing drilling of the lower clivus (LC). BA, basilar artery; PCICA, paraclival internal carotid artery.

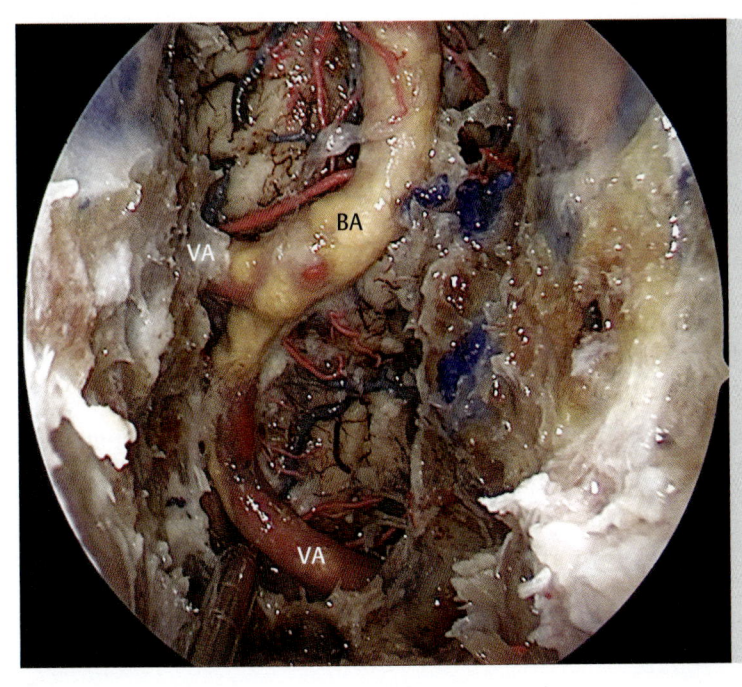

Fig. 7.46 Endoscopic image showing both the vertebral arteries (VA) uniting to form the basilar artery (BA).

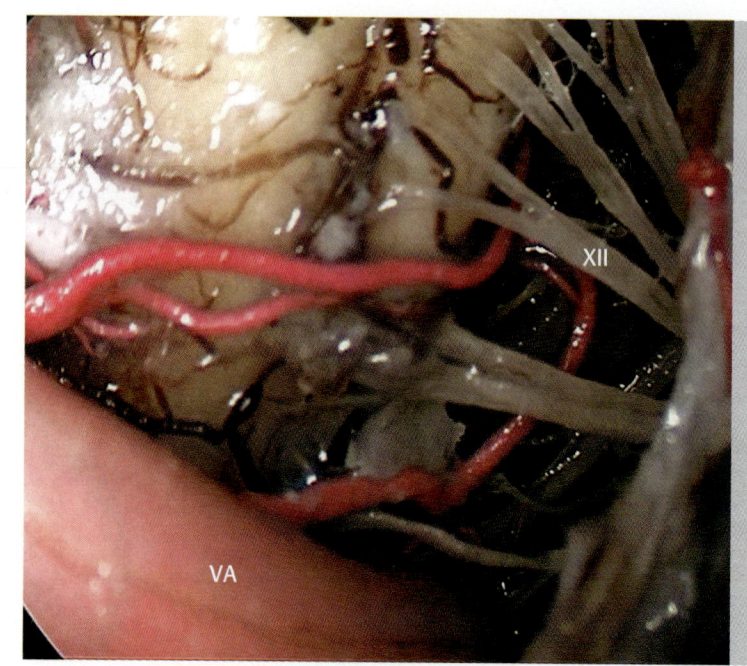

Fig. 7.47 Endoscopic image showing hypoglossal nerve (XII) and vertebral artery (VA).

which can be placed as interlay, or onlay graft. The vascularized pedicle graft is placed, and the edges are covered by Surgicel. If the defect is large or when the third ventricle is open a "gasket seal closure,"[14] this technique is preferred. This type of reconstruction includes a layer of soft tissue such as fascia lata placed in onlay plane covering the entire defect. Next, a piece of rigid material such as septal bone cartilage is fashioned to the size of bony defect. Then the solid graft is centered over the soft tissue graft as the soft tissue graft is present circumferentially around the rigid graft. The rigid graft is then pushed inside forming a gasket seal. The vascularized pedicle flap is placed over it. Care should be taken to ensure that the flap is in contact with bare bone all around its edges (**Fig. 7.48**).

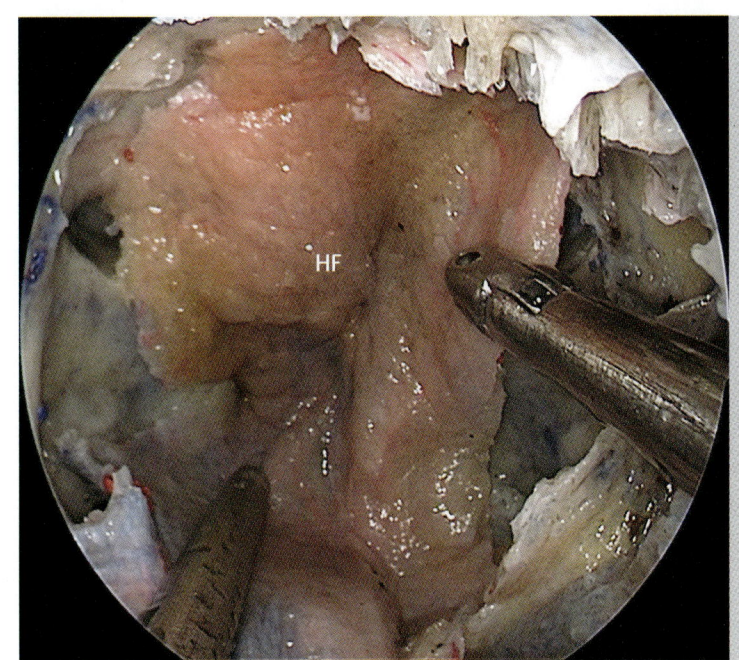

Fig. 7.48 Endoscopic image showing nasoseptal Hadad flap (HF) used to entirely cover the defect.

References

1. Price JC, Loury M, Carson B, Johns ME. The pericranial flap for reconstruction of anterior skull base defects. Laryngoscope 1988;98(11):1159–1164

2. Bent J, Kuhn FA, Cuilty C. The frontal cell in frontal recess obstruction. Am J Rhinol 1994;8:185–191

3. Bolger WE, Butzin CA, Parsons DS. Paranasal sinus bony anatomic variations and mucosal abnormalities: CT analysis for endoscopic sinus surgery. Laryngoscope 1991;101(1 Pt 1, 1pt 1):56–64

4. Lang J. Clinical Anatomy of the Nose, Nasal Cavity and Paranasal Sinuses. New York, NY: Thieme Medical Publishers; 1989:1–3

5. Fujii K, Chambers SM, Rhoton AL Jr. Neurovascular relationships of the sphenoid sinus. A microsurgical study. J Neurosurg 1979;50(1):31–39

6. Osawa S, Rhoton AL Jr, Tanriover N, Shimizu S, Fujii K. Microsurgical and surgical exposure. Neurosurgery 2008;63:210–238

7. Rhoton AL Jr. The posterior cranial fossa. Microsurgical anatomy and surgical approach. Neurosurgery 2006;47(3, Supp):S1–S298

8. Lang J. Anatomy of Nose, Nasal Cavity and Paranasal Sinus. New York, NY; Thieme Medical Publishers; 1989

9. Kassam AB, Gardner PA, Snyderman CH, Carrau RL, Mintz AH, Prevedello DM. Expanded endonasal approach, a fully endoscopic transnasal approach for the resection of midline suprasellar craniopharyngiomas: a new classification based on the infundibulum. J Neurosurg 2008;108(4):715–728

10. Kassam AB, Prevedello DM, Thomas A, et al. Endoscopic endonasal pituitary transposition for a transdorsum sellae approach to the interpeduncular cistern. Neurosurgery 2008; 62(3, Suppl 1):57–72, discussion 72–74

11. Lang J. Skull Base and Related Structures: Atlas of Clinical Anatomy. Stuttgart, Germany: Schattauer Verlag; 1995

12. Iaconetta G, Fusco M, Cavallo LM, Cappabianca P, Samii M, Tschabitscher M. The abducens nerve: microanatomic and endoscopic study. Neurosurgery 2007;61(3, Suppl):7–14, discussion 14

13. Kassam AB, Thomas A, Carrau RL, et al. Endoscopic reconstruction of the cranial base using a pedicled nasoseptal flap. Neurosurgery 2008;63(1, Suppl 1):ONS44–ONS52, discussion ONS52–ONS53

14. Leng LZ, Brown S, Anand VK, Schwartz TH. "Gasket-seal" watertight closure in minimal-access endoscopic cranial base surgery. Neurosurgery 2008;62(5, Suppl 2): E342–E343, discussion E343

08 Endoscopic Approaches in Coronal Plane

Narayanan Janakiram, Dharambir S. Sethi, Onkar K. Deshmukh, and Arvindh K. Gananathan

- § Introduction 157
- § Anterior Coronal Plane 158
- § Middle Coronal Plane 166
- § Posterior Coronal Approach 193
- § Conclusion 193

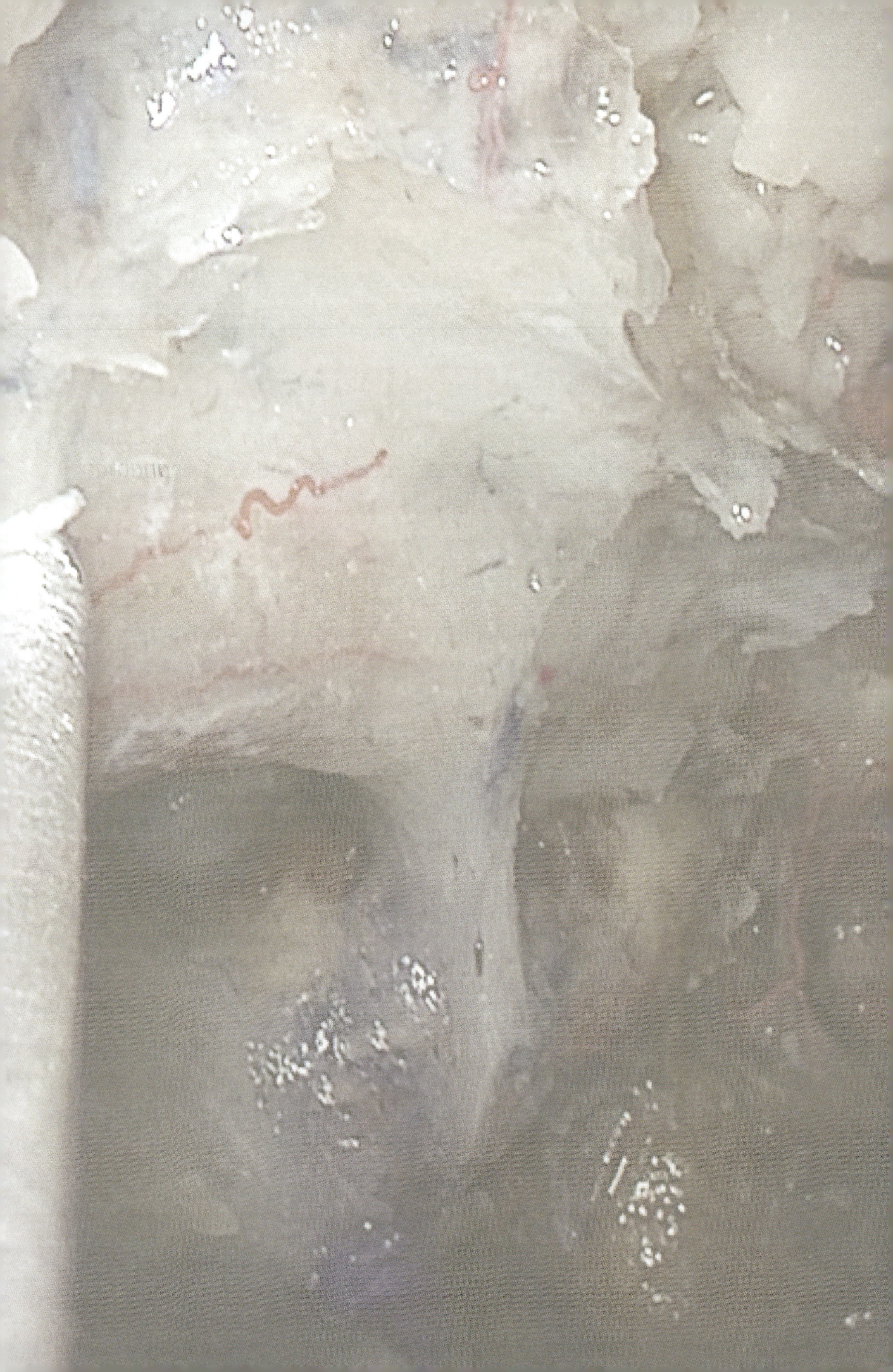

Introduction

Approaches in coronal plane are surgical trajectories to access anatomical subunits along the coronal planes of the ventral skull base. These can be roughly divided into anterior coronal plane including supra- and transorbital approaches; the middle coronal planes including the transpterygoid, transcavernous, and suprapetrous approaches; and finally, the posterior coronal approaches including the infrapetrous and parapharyngeal approaches.[1]

The anatomical subunits in the anterior coronal plane can be accessed directly by a homolateral endonasal endoscopic route; however, the surgical trajectories for the middle and posterior coronal planes pass through the maxillary sinus (transmaxillary). Thus, a partial endoscopic maxillectomy is a prerequisite for these approaches. Depending on the degree of lateral control desired, an endoscopic medial maxillectomy or a modified endoscopic Denker's approach is performed and a transmaxillary route is created for these approaches.

This chapter elaborates fundamental steps for dissection along various important approaches in all the three coronal planes (**Table 8.1**). It is of vital

Table 8.1 Approaches in coronal planes

	Approach	Areas accessed
Anterior coronal planes	Endonasal orbital decompression	Orbit
	Endonasal optic nerve decompression	Optic canal and nerve
Middle coronal planes	Transpterygoid approach to PPF/ITF	PPF, ITF
	Transpterygoid suprapetrous approach to Meckel's cave/inferior cavernous sinus	IOF, Meckel's cave, cavernous sinus
	Transpterygoid approach to superior cavernous sinus	Quadrangular space, superior cavernous sinus
Posterior coronal planes	Infrapetrous transpterygoid approach	Petrous apex bone

Abbreviations: IOF, inferior orbital fissure; ITF, infratemporal fossa; PPF, pterygopalatine fossa.

importance for the dissector to have a thorough knowledge of the intricate anatomy and three-dimensional orientation of the topography of skull base to mitigate the difficulties along the steep learning curve involved.

Anterior Coronal Plane

Orbital and Optic Nerve Decompression (Video 13)

The orbit and optic canal are confined to bony cavities, and any change in pressure owing to edema, tumor, or hemorrhage can cause rapid compromise on visual acuity and extraocular movements. Endoscopic endonasal approach to the orbit

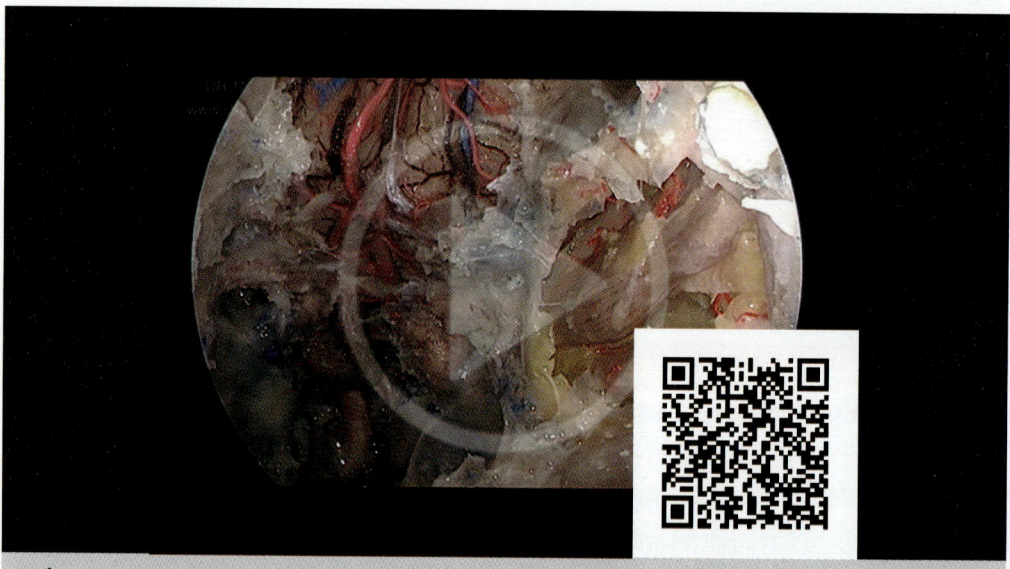

Video 13 Optic nerve and orbital decompression. https://www.thieme.de/de/q.htm?p=opn/tp/388257077/9789388257060_c001_v013&t=video

provides easy and safe access to these structures and provides better surgical outcomes. Orbital tumors medial to the neural axis and globe are amendable by this approach those lateral need an external approach or a transorbital corridor. This chapter focuses on endoscopic transnasal approach.

Relevant Anatomy

The nasal cavity and orbit are separated by a thin papery lateral bony wall of the ethmoid sinus, the lamina papyracea. The anterior and posterior ethmoidal arteries originate from the ophthalmic artery and traverse the roof of the orbit approximately 24 and 36 mm from the anterior lacrimal crest respectively.[2] The posterior ethmoidal artery is about 6 mm from the optic canal and lies 2 to 8 mm anterior to the anterior wall of the sphenoid sinus.

The optic canal is a cylindrical tunnel present between the lesser wing and body of the sphenoid bone that transmits optic nerve and ophthalmic artery. This oblique canal connects the cranial cavity and the orbit, and it opens on either side in the optic foramen. The point in the optic canal corresponding to the junction between the posterior ethmoid and sphenoid sinuses is the narrowest point in the canal. This is the site of attachment of the dura mater to the orbital periosteum, and the ligament of Zinn is also located at the same site. The ligament of Zinn or Zinn's annulus is fibrous where the tendons of the extraocular muscles merge at the apex of the orbit.

Proximally along the course of the optic nerve, the ophthalmic artery lies inferolaterally to the nerve. Proceeding distally along the optic canal, its orientation changes to inferomedial. This aspect should be considered while drilling the optic canal and incising the sheath of the optic nerve to prevent an inadvertent injury or rupture of this artery.

Orbital Decompression

Orbital decompression involves removal of one or more walls of the orbit. This is primarily performed to release the intraorbital pressure in cases of Grave's disease or in cases of orbital hemorrhage from the retracted anterior ethmoidal artery that is transected during functional endoscopic sinus surgery. This procedure may also be performed as an initial step during endonasal endoscopic transorbital approaches to the orbital apex.

Orbital decompression commences with a partial uncinectomy and wide middle meatal antrostomy. The maxillary sinus ostium is widened anteriorly till the nasolacrimal duct, inferiorly till the superior border of the inferior turbinate, superiorly till the orbital floor, and posteriorly till the posterior wall of the maxillary sinus. This is followed by anterior and posterior ethmoidectomy and a wide sphenoidectomy. The anterior wall of the sphenoid sinus is removed completely. Now with help of a Cottle's elevator and sickle knife, the lamina papyracea is removed from the junction of the lamina with the lacrimal bone till just anterior to the sphenoid sinus wall where Zinn's annulus is located (**Fig. 8.1**). Care is taken not to damage the periorbita. Now the bone of the floor of the orbit is removed till the canal of the infraorbital nerve. It is prudent to decompress the orbit along one and half of its walls to achieve adequate retrogression of the globe (**Fig. 8.2**).

On removal of the lamina papyracea, the orbital fat is seen and the dissector may carefully remove the fat exposing the medial rectus muscle (**Fig. 8.3**). Similarly, the inferior and superior recti and the superior oblique muscles are identified. The trajectories between the inferior and medial rectus and superior oblique and medial rectus are used to approach the orbital apex lesions (**Fig. 8.4**).[3]

Endoscopic Approaches in Coronal Plane

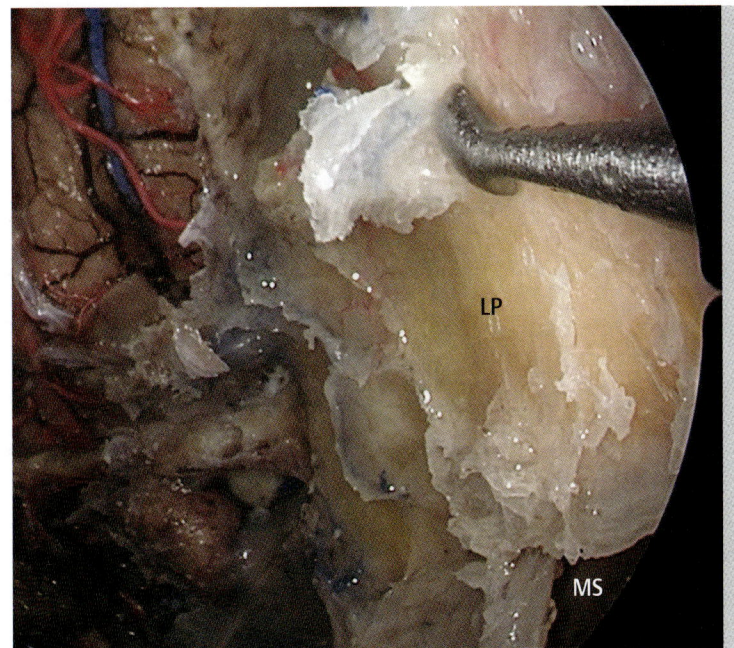

Fig. 8.1 Endoscopic image showing removal of lamina papyracea from the medial wall of the orbit. LP, lamina papyracea; MS, maxillary sinus.

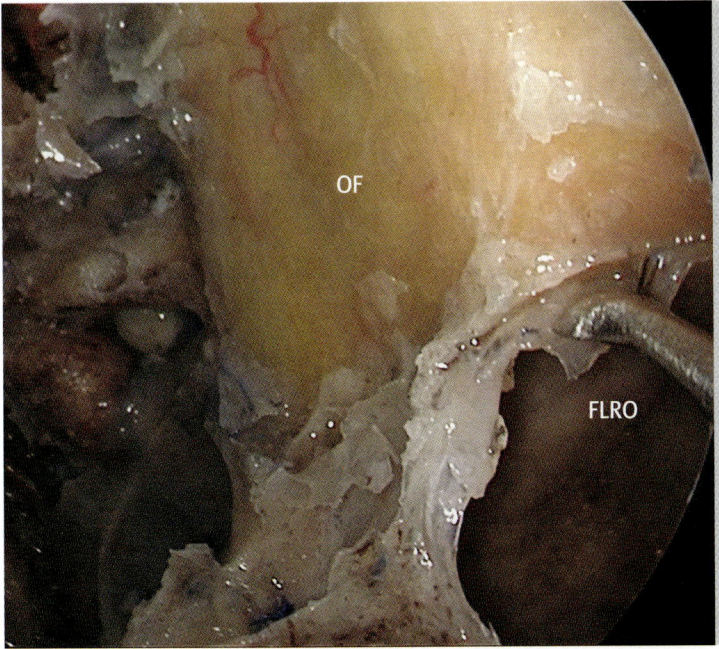

Fig. 8.2 Endoscopic image showing removal of floor of the orbit till the infraorbital nerve canal. OF, orbital fat; FLRO, floor of orbit.

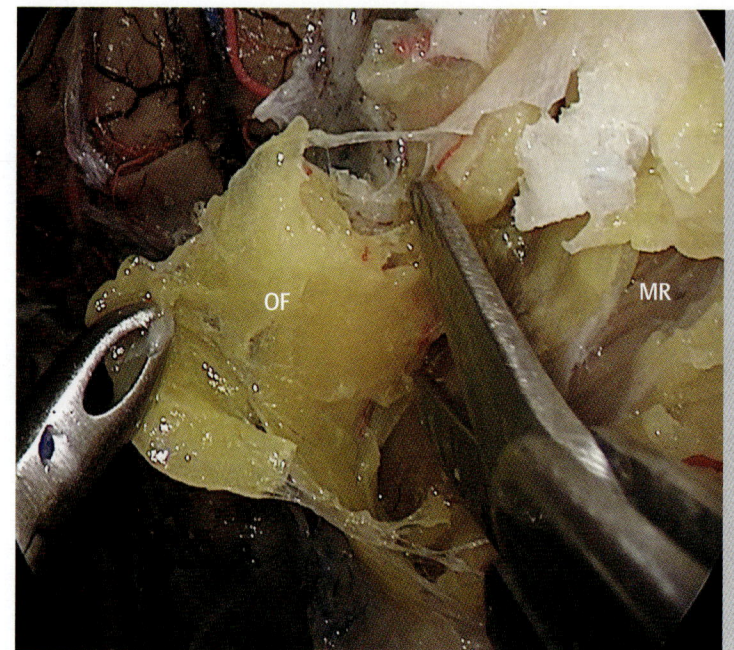

Fig. 8.3 Endoscopic image showing removal of the orbital fat till exposure of medial rectus. OF, orbital fat; MR, medial rectus.

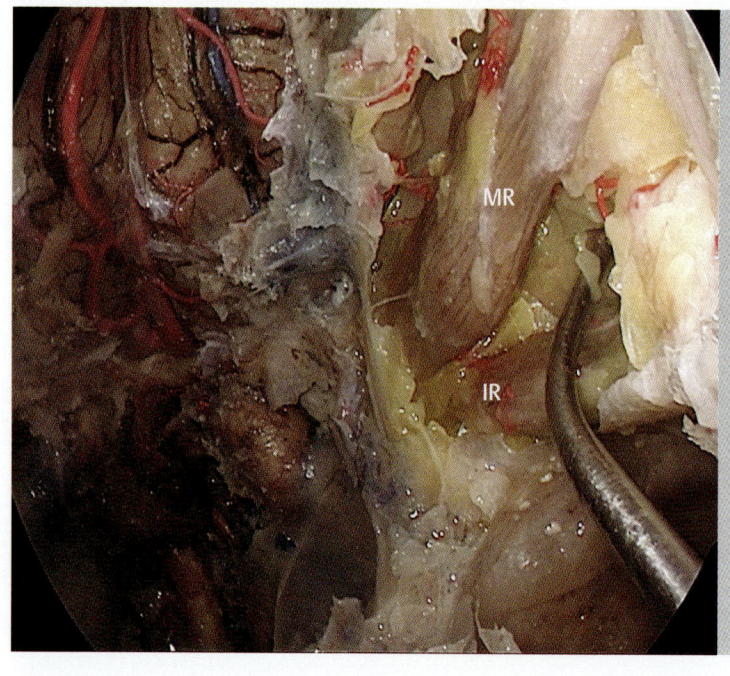

Fig. 8.4 Endoscopic image showing ball probe placed in transorbital approach to orbital apex. IR, inferior rectus; MR, medial rectus.

Optic Nerve Decompression

Optic nerve decompression involves removing a part of the bone of the optic canal all along its length in order to relieve the pressure on the optic nerve caused due to traumatic edema or due to nonosseous lesions or pseudotumor cerebri leading to comprised vision. Other rare causes are mucoceles of sphenoid sinus, schwannomas, and NAION (nonarteritic anterior ischemic neuropathy).

The procedure begins as uni-nostril two-handed approach with a 0-degree endoscope. A partial uncinectomy, middle meatal antrostomy, anterior and posterior ethmoidectomy, and a wide sphenoidectomy are performed. The entire anterior wall of the sphenoid sinus is then removed with a Kerrison's punch or with a high-speed endonasal drill with a diamond burr. The impression of the optic canal is identified on the lateral and posterior wall of the sphenoid sinus. The decompression commences with a long intranasal drill with a diamond burr along the long axis of the optic nerve (**Fig. 8.5**). The ligament of Zinn is identified anteriorly, and the drilling proceeds posteriorly till the posterior wall of the sphenoid sinus (**Fig. 8.6**). Minimum circumferential decompression is 180 degrees around the entire length of the nerve. A curette is used to chip out the thin layer of the bone over the nerve (**Fig. 8.7**). Once the entire bony canal is drilled from the posterior wall of the sphenoid to the Zinn's annulus and the medial rectus anteriorly, a sickle knife or a no. 15 blade is used to incise the nerve sheath. The incision is taken in the superomedial quadrant (between 12- and 3-o' clock on the right side and between 9- and 12-o' clock on the left). Care should be taken not to injure the ophthalmic artery while incising the nerve sheath (**Fig. 8.8**).

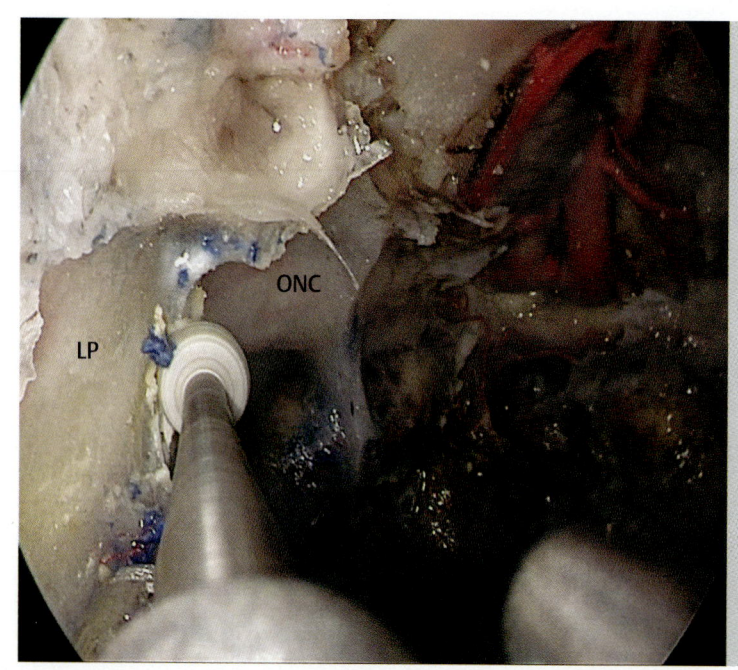

Fig. 8.5 Endoscopic image showing commencement of drilling at the annulus of Zinn for decompression of the optic nerve. LP, lamina papyracea; ONC, optic nerve canal.

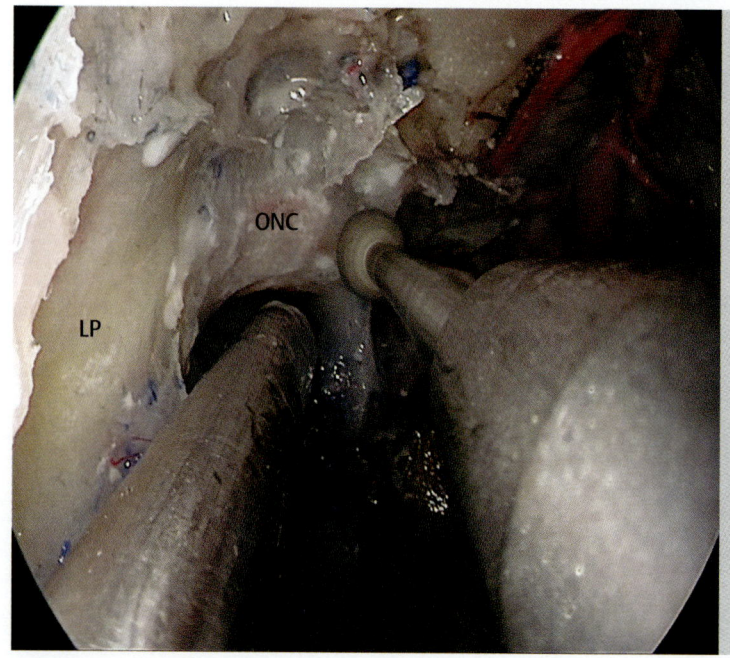

Fig. 8.6 Endoscopic image showing the decompression along the axis of optic nerve in an anteroposterior direction. LP, lamina papyracea; ONC, optic nerve canal.

Endoscopic Approaches in Coronal Plane

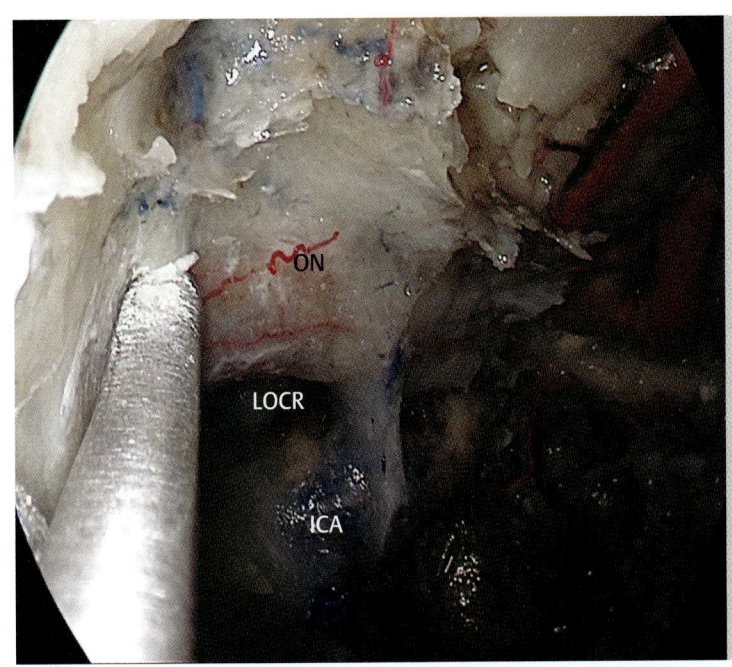

Fig. 8.7 Endoscopic image showing removal of small chips of bone with Cottle's elevator. ICA, internal carotid artery; LOCR, lateral optic carotid recess; ON, optic nerve.

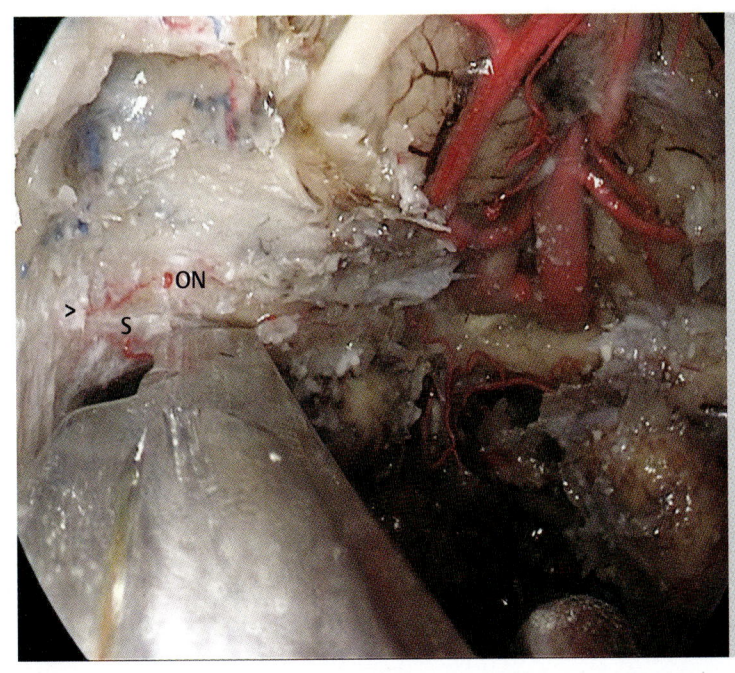

Fig. 8.8 Endoscopic image showing incision over dural sheath of optic nerve. ON, optic nerve; S, nerve sheath; >, incision.

Middle Coronal Plane

Access through Maxillary Sinus—Endoscopic Endonasal Transmaxillary Approaches

In ventral skull base surgery, endoscopic trajectory to access lesions occupying the anatomical subunits in the coronal plane should primarily pass through the maxillary sinus. Depending on the location or lateral extent of the lesion, transmaxillary approaches such as endoscopic medial maxillectomy or endoscopic modified Denker's approach are preferred. These two transmaxillary approaches provide progressively better lateral control of dissection.[4]

Endoscopic Medial Maxillectomy

The dissection begins as a uni-nostril two-handed approach with a 0-degree endoscope. A partial uncinectomy, wide middle meatal antrostomy with anterior-posterior ethmoidectomy, and sphenoidotomy are performed. The antrostomy extends till the lacrimal bone anteriorly, caudally till the upper end of the inferior turbinate, and superiorly till the orbital floor. Posteriorly it extends till the posterior wall of the maxillary sinus. Now with turbinectomy scissors, the inferior turbinate is resected along its lateral attachment (**Fig. 8.9**). With a debrider or a Weil Blakesley straight forceps, the mucosa of the inferior meatus corresponding to the remnant medial wall of the maxillary sinus inferiorly is removed. This exposed bone of the medial wall is now removed with a rongeur or a high-speed drill having a cutting burr. Hereby the entire medial wall of the maxilla is completely resected.

This exposure provides access to the medial part of the posterior maxillary wall and the pterygoid complex. Its lateral access can be augmented by creating a septal window and adopting the bi-nostril four-handed approach. A septal window is created by removing a small piece of septal cartilage anterior to the anterior

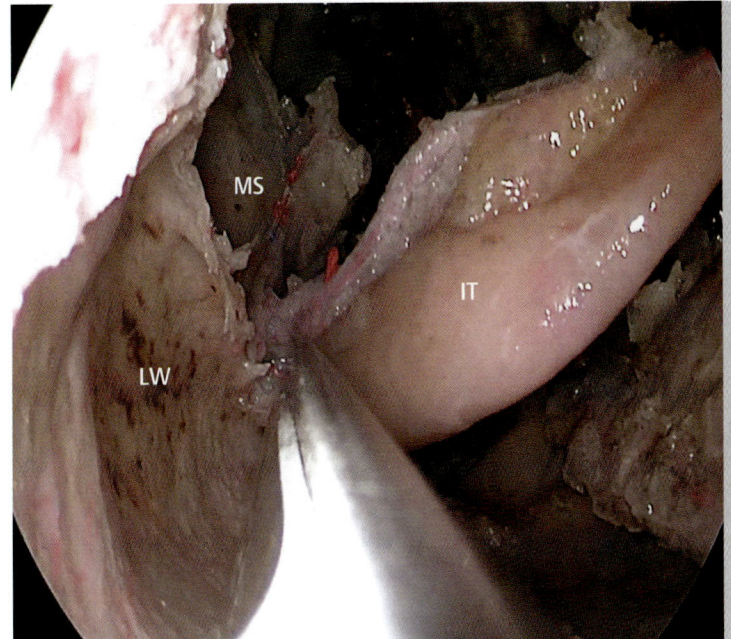

Fig. 8.9 Endoscopic image showing inferior turbinate resection. IT, inferior turbinate; LW, lateral wall; MS, maxillary sinus.

end of the middle turbinate through perpendicular incisions (vertical on left and horizontal on the right sides of septal mucoperichondrium) on both sides of septal mucoperichondria. Now an instrument may be manipulated through the passage, thus created from the opposite nostril of the maxillectomy.

Endoscopic Modified Denker's Procedure (Video 14)

Similar to a medial maxillectomy, the Denker's procedure also commences with a partial uncinectomy, wide middle meatal antrostomy, anterior-posterior ethmoidectomy, and a wide sphenoidotomy. The inferior turbinate is resected, and the mucosa over the lateral wall of the inferior meatus is removed. Now with a knife, the mucoperiosteum over the lower part pyriform aperture is incised. With a Cottle's elevator, a periosteal flap is elevated laterally over the anterior wall of the maxilla (**Fig. 8.10**). The elevation is extended posterosuperiorly until the infraorbital

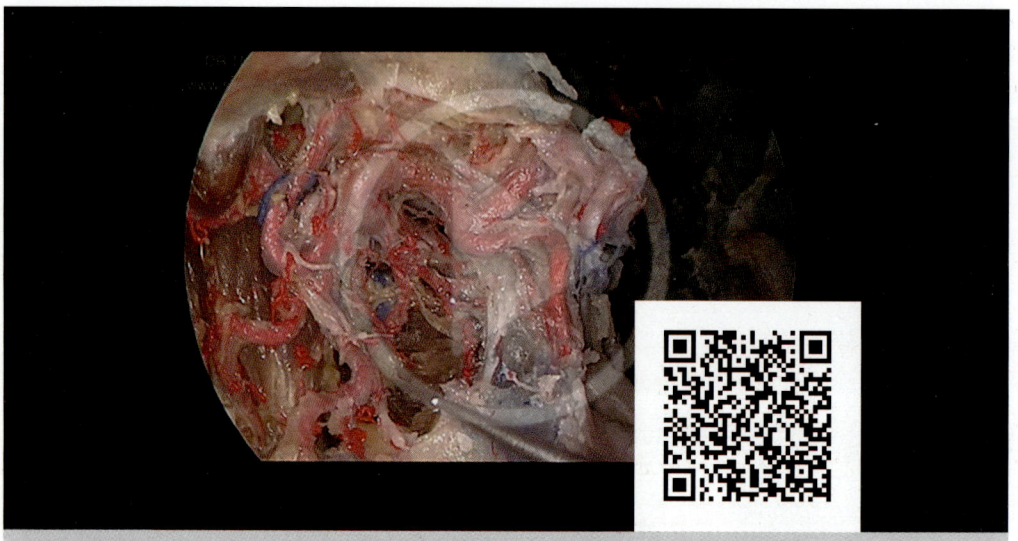

Video 14 Endoscopic endonasal transmaxillary approach (endoscopic modified Denker's procedure and approach to pterygopalatine fossa). https://www.thieme.de/de/q.htm?p=opn/tp/388257077/9789388257060_c001_v014&t=video

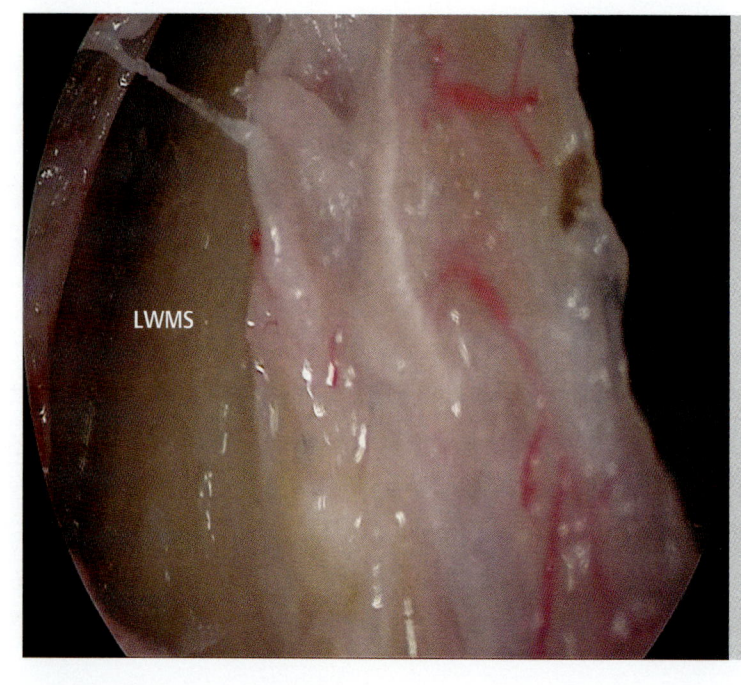

Fig. 8.10 Endoscopic image showing elevation of lateral periosteal flap from the pyriform aperture. LWMS, lateral wall of maxillary sinus.

Endoscopic Approaches in Coronal Plane

nerve canal is visualized. Now with an assistant retracting the flap laterally, a four-handed bimanual approach is adopted. The assistant holds the scope, and the dissector uses the drill and suction through the same nostril (**Fig. 8.11**). The maxillary sinus cavity is entered drilling through its anterior wall. The aperture created is now widened superiorly till the roof of the maxillary sinus and inferiorly to the floor of the maxillary sinus, and corresponding part of the pyriform aperture is also drilled out (**Fig. 8.12**). As the drilling proceeds posteriorly along the medial wall, the nasolacrimal duct is encountered. The bone around the duct is removed, and the duct is transected with sharp scissors (**Fig. 8.13**). The entire medial wall of the maxillary sinus until the posterior wall is drilled out. Following this, the mucosa over the posterior wall of the maxillary sinus is removed with a Blakesley forceps.

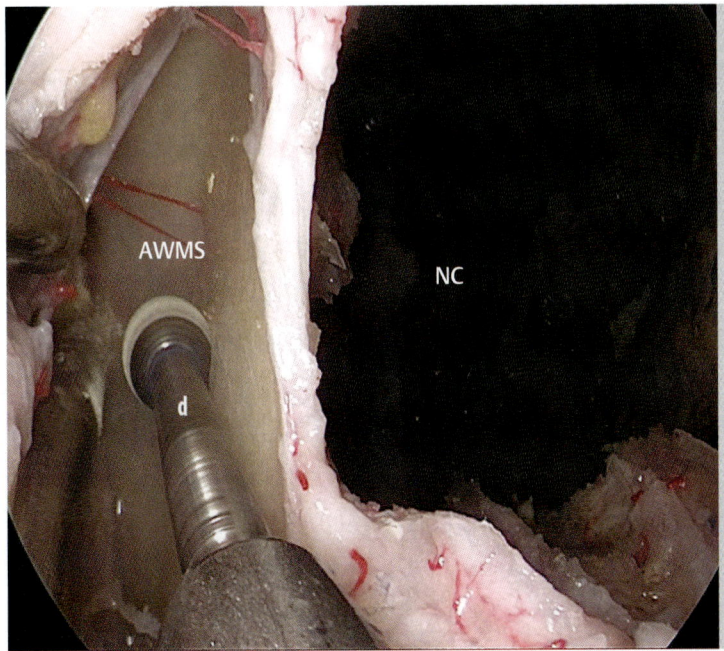

Fig. 8.11 Endoscopic image showing complete exposure for Denker's. Note the posterosuperior limit the infraorbital canal. AWMS, anterior wall of maxillary sinus; NC, nasal cavity.

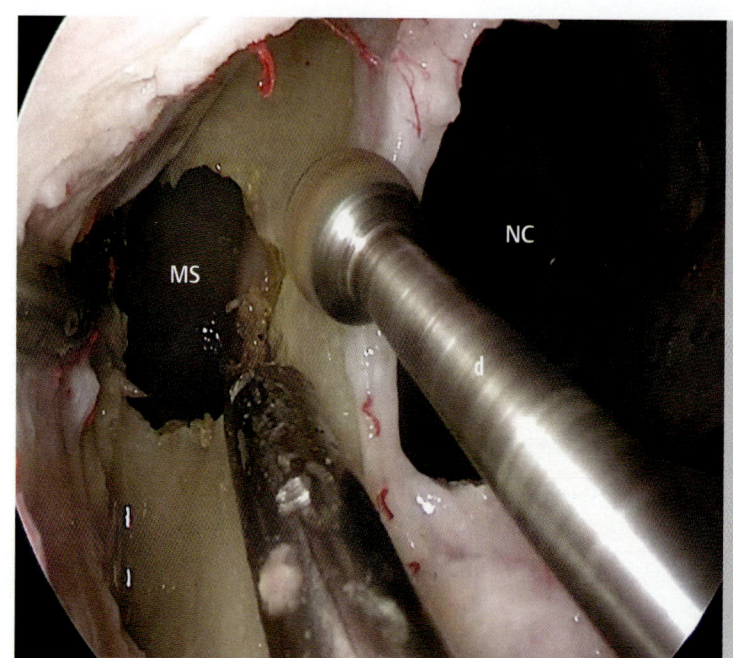

Fig. 8.12 Endoscopic image showing the maxillary antrum after drilling the anterior wall. MS, maxillary sinus; NC, nasal cavity.

Transpterygoid Approach to Pterygopalatine Fossa

The pterygopalatine fossa (PPF) houses a number of neurovascular structures relaying them to various cavities that it connects. The endoscopic approach has provided excellent visibility and safe and easy access to the PPF. It is accessed for purpose of ligation of the internal maxillary artery (IMA) in patients in whom ligation of the sphenopalatine artery (SPA) has failed or for vidian neurectomy in patients with refractory vasomotor rhinitis. Also, tumors such as juvenile nasopharyngeal angiofibroma (JNA) and maxillary nerve schwannomas originate in the vicinity of PPF, and so the PPF needs to be exposed to access these tumors. More commonly, the PPF needs to be exposed to gain access via the transpterygoid approaches to cavernous sinus, Meckel's cave, and infratemporal fossa (ITF).

Endoscopic Approaches in Coronal Plane

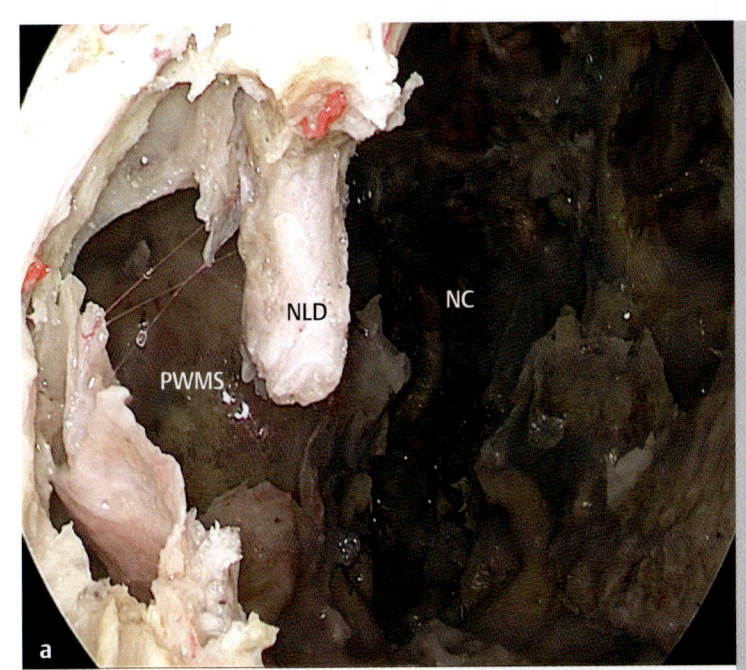

Fig. 8.13 Endoscopic image showing **(a)** complete exposure after modified endoscopic Denker's procedure and **(b)** transection of the nasolacrimal duct with scissors. NLD, nasolacrimal duct; PWMS, posterior wall of maxillary sinus.

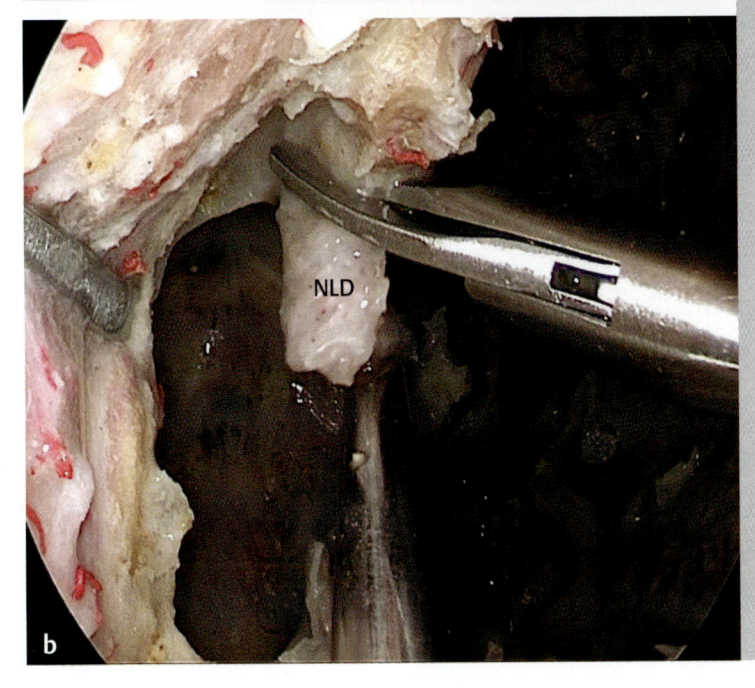

Relevant Anatomy

The PPF is an inverted pyramidal-shaped space located between the posterior wall of the maxillary sinus and base of pterygoid process. It opens laterally in the ITF via the pterygomaxillary fissure and communicates with the nasal cavity by the sphenopalatine foramen that transmits the SPA and nerves. The inferior orbital fissure connects it to the orbit and transmits the infraorbital and zygomatic branches of the maxillary nerve, infraorbital artery, and a branch of the inferior ophthalmic vein. Its anterior wall is formed by the posterior wall of maxillary sinus and superiorly by the orbital process of palatine bone. The superior wall of the fossa corresponds to the lower border of greater wing of sphenoid and the floor or sphenoid sinus. The medial wall of the PPF is formed by the vertical lamina of the palatine bone, and it articulates with the posterior wall of maxillary sinus anteriorly. At its junction posteriorly with the medial pterygoid process, it forms the sphenopalatine foramen. The lamina of the medial wall divides into two processes at its upper end. The first process fuses to form the superomedial part of the maxillary antrum. The second process is thinner, and with the pterygoid canal it forms the pterygopalatine or the palatovaginal canal.

Lateral to its medial wall, the PPF forms the greater palatine canal that continues to its apex inferiorly to communicate with the oral cavity through the greater palatine foramen. This transmits the greater palatine nerves and vessels (descending palatine artery [DPA]).

The PPF consists of fat, the pterygopalatine ganglion, vidian nerve, V2 or maxillary division, or the trigeminal nerve and the branches of the third part of the IMA. The blood vessels and the fat lie anterior to the neural structures and thus are encountered first in the endoscopic approach.

The V2 or the maxillary division of the trigeminal nerve enters the PPF posteriorly through the foramen rotundum. This nerve communicates with the pterygopalatine ganglion and gives branches to the orbit via inferior orbital fissure and to the nasal cavity.

The ITF lies in lateral relation to the PPF. It is laterally bounded by the ramus of the mandible and the pterygoid muscles. Its roof is formed by the greater wing of the sphenoid bone and posteriorly lies the articular tubercle of the temporal bone and spine of the sphenoid. Medially it communicates with the PPF and transmits the IMA via the pterygomaxillary fissure. The IMA is one of the terminal branches of the external carotid artery and is divided into three parts by the lateral pterygoid muscle. The third part of this artery traverses initially vertically and then horizontally along the ITF and PPF. Its terminal branches are the SPA and DPA. Other branches are namely the infraorbital artery, posterosuperior alveolar artery, and artery of the pterygoid canal. The artery of the pterygoid canal can have its origin from the IMA or ICA. This artery is a content of the pterygoid canal along with the pterygoid nerve or the vidian nerve (formed by greater superficial petrosal nerve and deep petrosal nerve). This supplies autonomic fibers to the lacrimal gland. This canal is one of the most important landmarks for the anterior genu of the ICA.[5]

Dissection of the Pterygopalatine Fossa (Video 14)

Initially, a medial maxillectomy or a modified Denker's approach is performed. The PPF is accessed by a bi-nostril four-handed approach with a 0-degree endoscope in the same nostril as that of the fossa to be approached. The suction is always introduced in the right nostril and instrument in the left, and using the septal window, both are brought on the side to be operated. The medial edge of the posterior wall is exposed and the SPA identified at the crista ethmoidale (**Fig. 8.14**). The mucosa over the posterior wall of the maxillary sinus is removed with a Blakesley forceps. With a high-speed drill or a punch, the posterior wall of the maxillary sinus is removed (**Fig. 8.15**). The limits of the resection are laterally till the junction of the lateral and the posterior wall, medially till the perpendicular

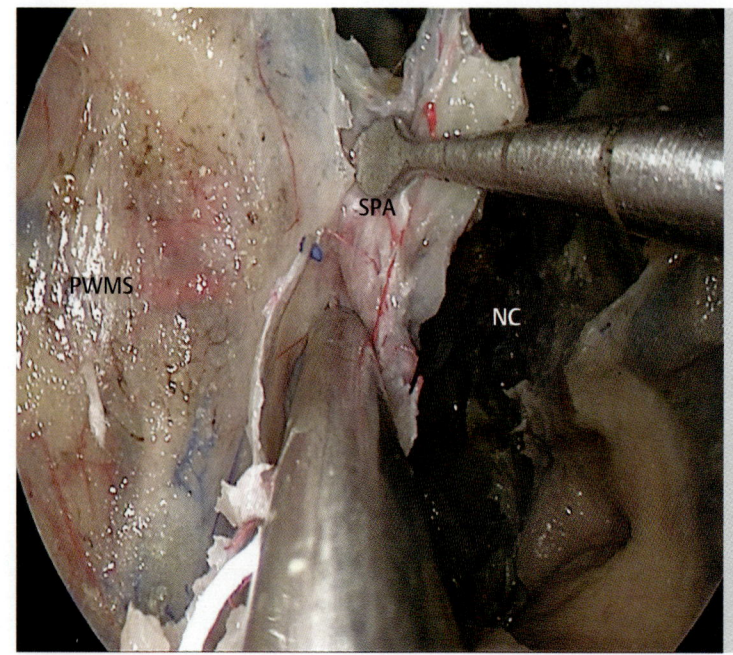

Fig. 8.14 Endoscopic image showing sphenopalatine artery (SPA) arising at crista ethmoidale medial edge of the posterior wall of maxillary sinus (PWMS). NC, nasal cavity.

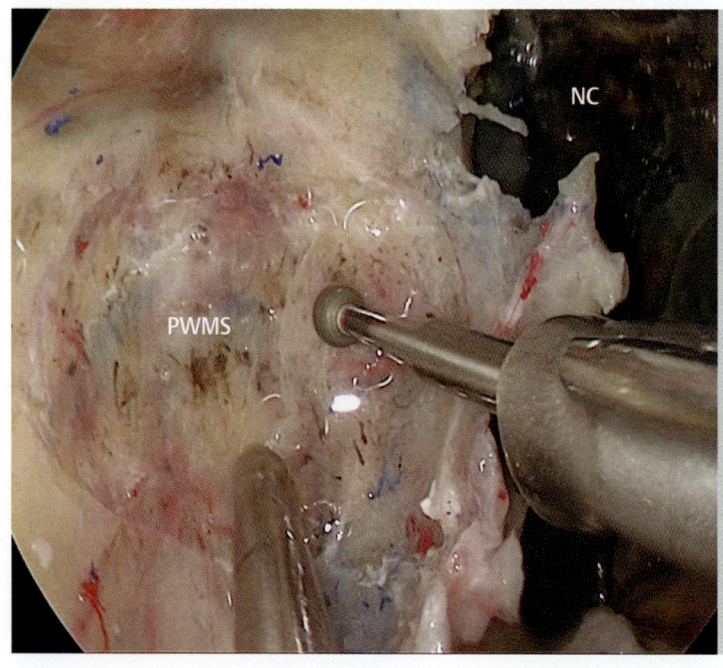

Fig. 8.15 Endoscopic image showing removal of posterior wall of maxillary sinus (PWMS). NC, nasal cavity.

plate of palatine bone, and superiorly till the orbital process of palatine bone. After the bony wall is removed, the periosteum behind the posterior wall is exposed. The periosteum is incised such that the arteries just posterior to it are not injured. Fine scissors are used for this purpose (**Fig. 8.16**).

The sagittal plane passing through the lateral pterygoid plate divides the posterior wall of the maxilla into a medial PPF and a lateral ITF. The pterygomaxillary fissure area is dissected, and a debrider or Blakesley forceps laterally removes the fat protruding out. The branches of the third part of the IMA are identified. The SPA and DPA are the two terminal branches of the IMA. The SPA is traced from the sphenopalatine foramen backward to find the main trunk, and the other branches are dissected subsequently (**Fig. 8.17**). The main trunk is followed proximally in between the two heads of the lateral pterygoid muscle (**Fig. 8.18**). The SPA and DPA are clipped and divided. Following this, the infraorbital nerve is dissected along the

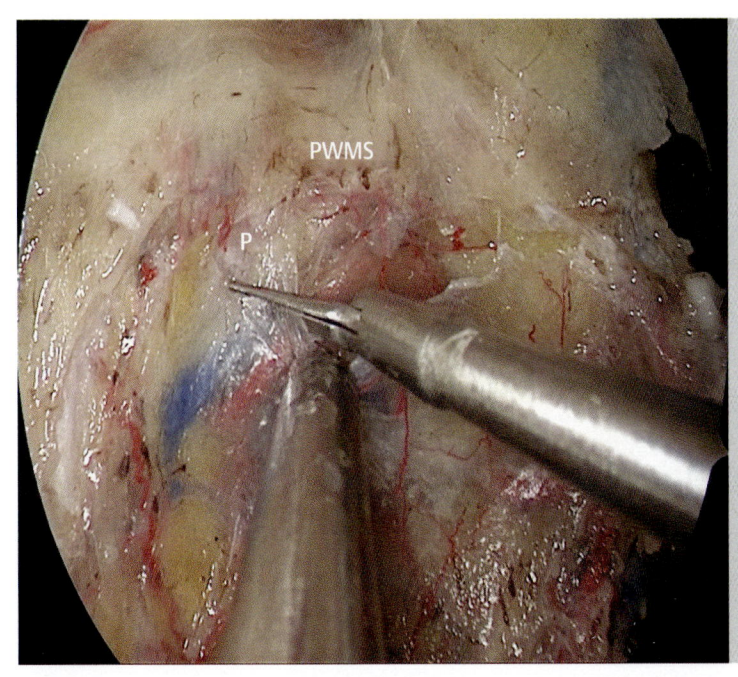

Fig. 8.16 Endoscopic image showing incising the periosteum (P) over pterygopalatine fossa and infratemporal fossa with fine scissors. PWMS, posterior wall of maxillary sinus.

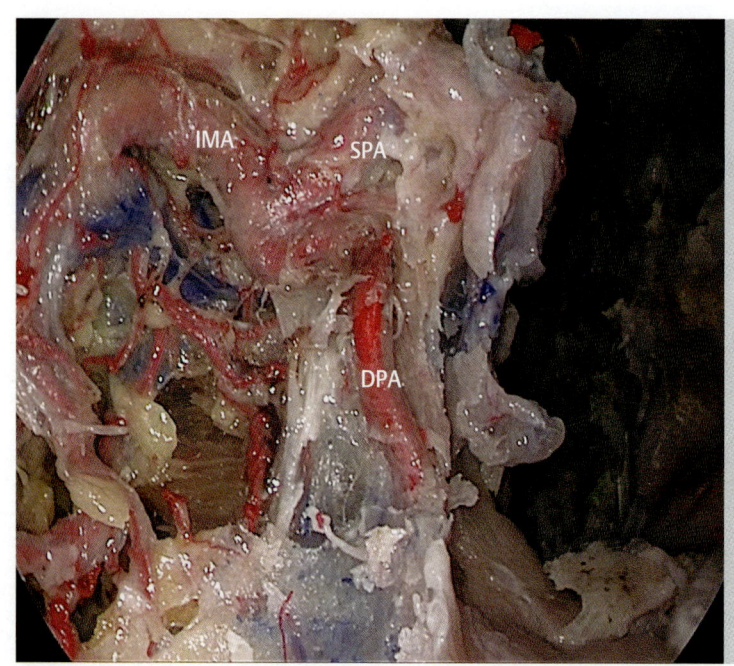

Fig. 8.17 Endoscopic image showing delineation of sphenopalatine artery (SPA) and descending palatine artery (DPA). IMA, internal maxillary artery.

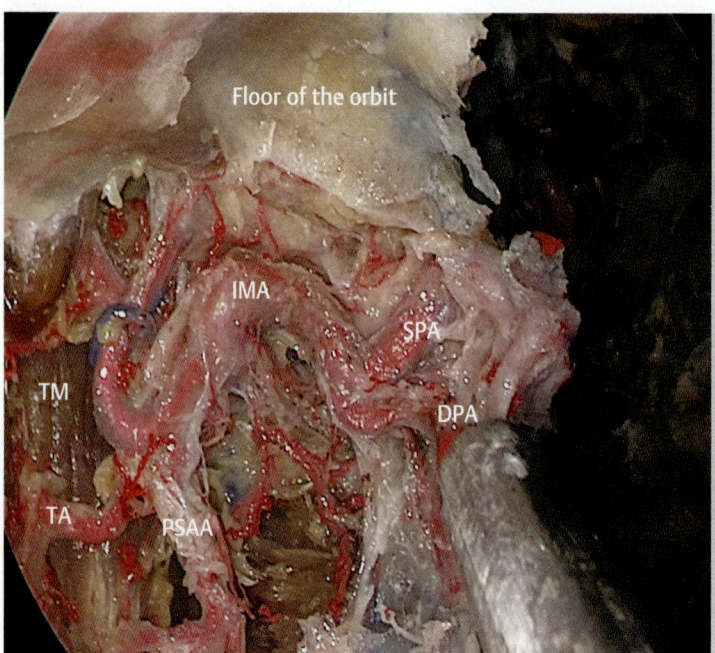

Fig. 8.18 Endoscopic image showing third part of internal maxillary artery with all its branches. DPA, descending palatine artery; IMA, internal maxillary artery; PSAA, posterior superior alveolar artery; SPA, sphenopalatine artery; TA, temporal artery; TM, temporalis muscle.

Endoscopic Approaches in Coronal Plane 177

superior margin of the PPF and is followed to trace the V2 back to the foramen rotundum. The contents of the PPF are retracted laterally to expose the pterygoid wedge or base. Drilling of this bone comprises transpterygoid approach.

Dissection of/Approach to Infratemporal Fossa (Video 15)

Lesions such as JNA, V2 schwannomas, and mucormycosis primarily enter the PPF and also extend to the ITF. Other lesions that encroach upon the ITF include V3 schwannomas, parapharyngeal tumor AV malformations, and hemangiomas. The ITF is safely accessed via the transpterygoid route. Such an access is also needed to internalize a temporoparietal flap for nasal reconstruction. A modified endoscopic Denker's approach is generally essential to obtain access to ITF.

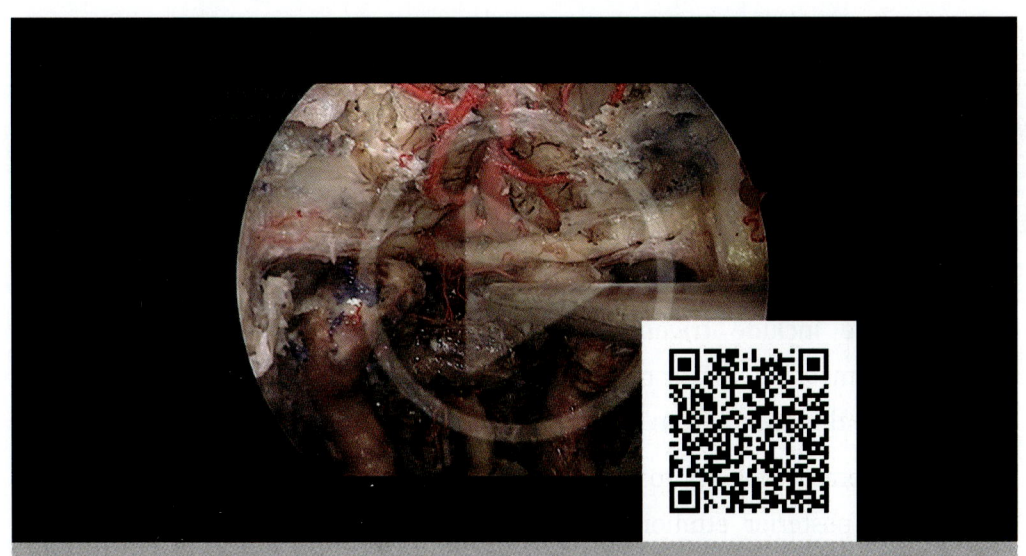

Video 15 Transpterygoid approach to cavernous sinus and approach to infratemporal fossa. https://www.thieme.de/de/q.htm?p=opn/tp/388257077/9789388257060_c001_v015&t=video

Dissection

Following exposure of the PPF by a modified endoscopic Denker's approach, the IMA is ligated and divided at the level of the lateral pterygoid muscle. The muscles in the ITF are identified, especially the medial pterygoid muscle. The primary content of the ITF is the mandibular nerve; the main trunk is identified just posterior to the root of the lateral pterygoid plate at its emergence from the foramen ovale. Following this, the two main branches of the posterior trunk of the mandibular nerve, the lingual and the inferior alveolar nerves, are identified. The middle meningeal artery is now identified arising posterior and lateral to the nerve from the foramen ovale (**Fig. 8.19**). The muscles are resected, and the pterygoid plexus of veins are identified and removed. Now the vertical fibers of the tensor palatini muscles are identified along the eustachian tube (ET) (**Fig. 8.20**). The medial part of the cartilaginous ET is now resected with angled scissors directed away from the carotid artery. This exposes the parapharyngeal carotid artery. The soft tissue over it is carefully removed completing the dissection of the ITF (**Fig. 8.21**).

Suprapetrous Transpterygoid Approach to the Meckel's Cave/Inferior Cavernous Sinus (Video 15)

Meckel's cave is dural diverticulum in the middle cranial fossa that houses the gasserian ganglion of the trigeminal nerve. The three divisions of the trigeminal nerve originate from the gasserian ganglion. Pathologies common to the Meckel's cave include trigeminal schwannomas, meningiomas, chondromas, chondrosarcomas, etc. A few others such as adenoid cystic carcinomas and JNAs also spread to this region from the nasal cavity.

The surprapetrous approach starts with a unilateral maxillary antrostomy, anterior and posterior ethmoidectomy, bilateral sphenoidectomy, and posterior septectomy. For the purpose of reconstruction, a contralateral Hadad flap is preferred.

Endoscopic Approaches in Coronal Plane

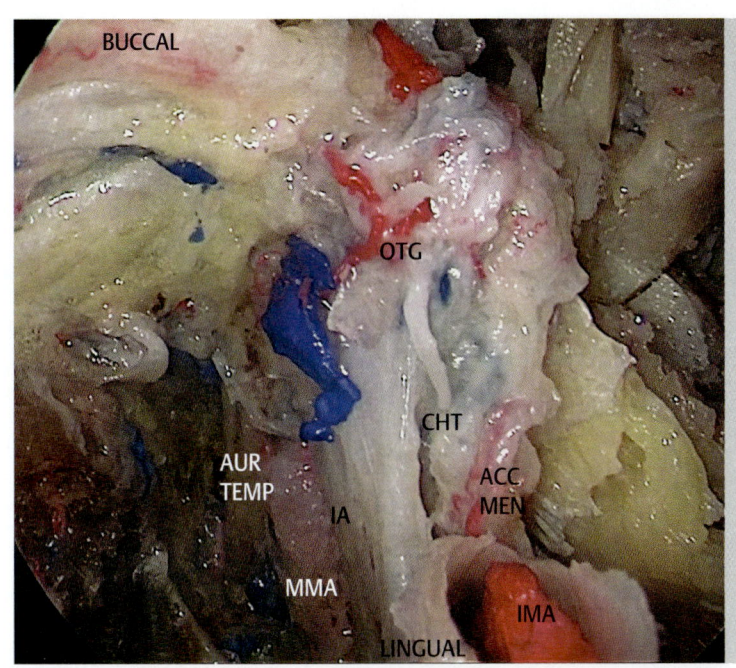

Fig. 8.19 Endoscopic image showing complete exposure of infratemporal fossa showing branches of the mandibular nerve. ACC MEN; AUR TEMP, auriculotemporal nerve; BUCCAL, buccal nerve; CHT; IMA, internal maxillary artery; IA, inferior alveolar nerve; LINGUAL, lingual nerve; MMA, middle meningeal artery; OTG, otic ganglion.

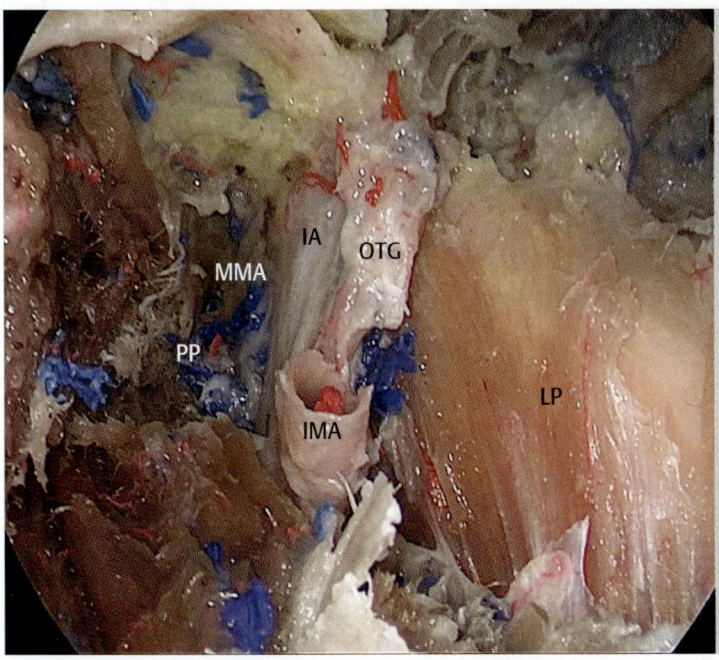

Fig. 8.20 Endoscopic image showing complete exposure of infratemporal fossa After removal of the muscles to reveal the Eustachian tube. IMA, internal maxillary artery; LP, lateral pterygoid plate; OTG, otic ganglion; IA, inferior alveolar artery; PP, pterygoid plexus; MMA, middle meningeal artery.

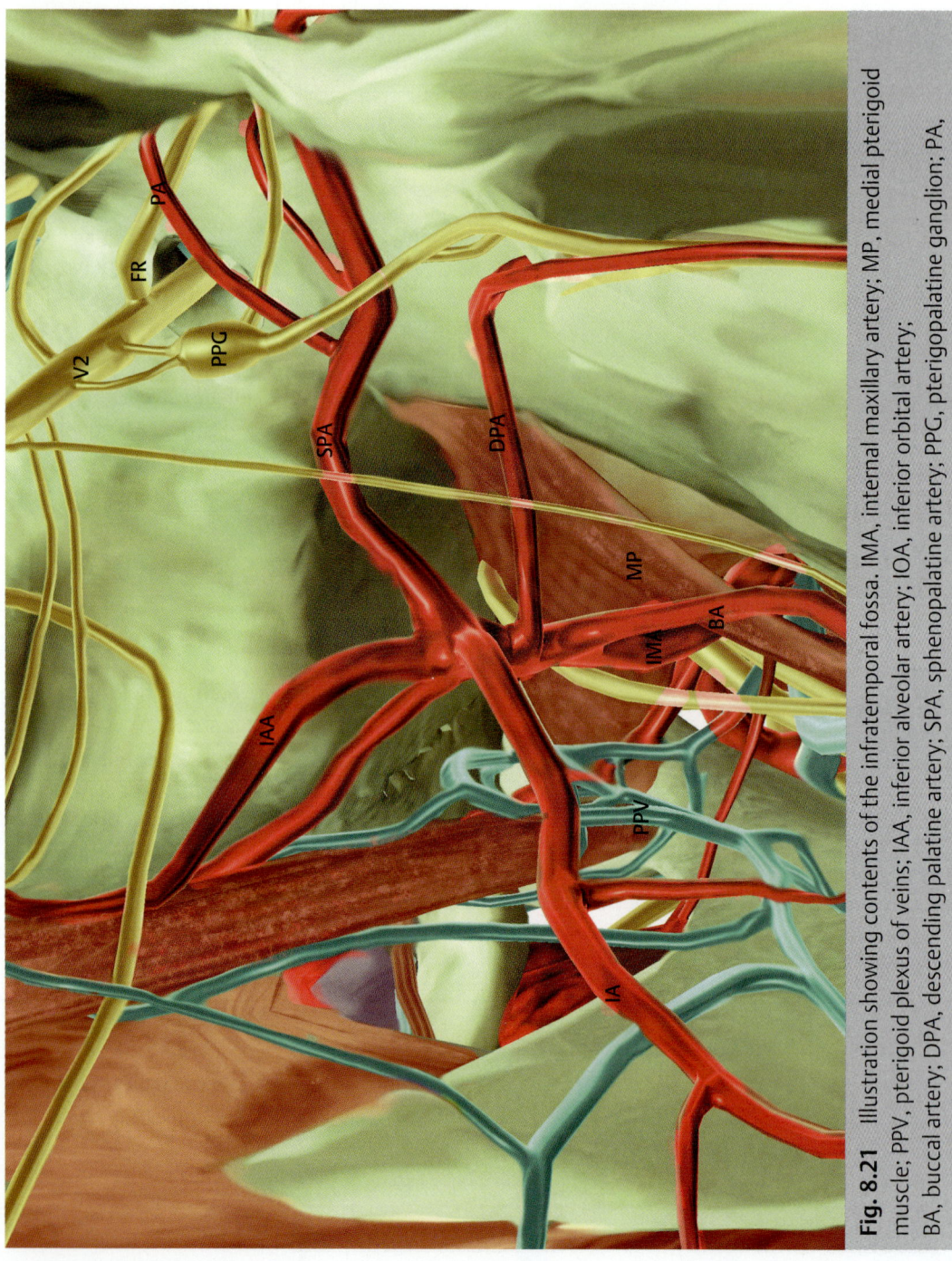

Fig. 8.21 Illustration showing contents of the infratemporal fossa. IMA, internal maxillary artery; MP, medial pterygoid muscle; PPV, pterygoid plexus of veins; IAA, inferior alveolar artery; IOA, inferior orbital artery; BA, buccal artery; DPA, descending palatine artery; SPA, sphenopalatine artery; PPG, pterygopalatine ganglion; PA, pharyngeal artery; FR, foramen rotundum; V2, maxillary division of trigeminal nerve.

Relevant Anatomy

The cavernous sinus is present on either side of the sella extending from superior orbital fissure to petrous part of the temporal bone. Several venous channels may connect both the cavernous sinus, namely superior, middle, inferior, and posterior intercavernous sinus. The cavernous sinus is divided into three main compartments by their relations with the carotid artery: the medial, anteroinferior, and posterosuperior (between carotid and posterior half of roof of sinus) compartment.

The dural covering of the cavernous sinus includes meningeal layers that cover the brain and form diaphragma sellae and endosteal that is the periosteum of sphenoid bone, which extends along the roof, posterior and lateral walls of the cavernous sinus. The lateral wall of cavernous sinus has two layers: meningeal and endosteal.

Medial wall of cavernous is divided into superior and inferior parts. The inferior part is covered by the endosteal layer of the dura toward the sphenoid bone and the superior part is covered by the meningeal layer of the dura over the sella.

The roof of the cavernous sinus is divided into two parts: anterior that has the clinoidal triangle and posterior that has the oculomotor triangle. The anterior petroclinoid fold connects between anterior clinoid and petrous apex. The posterior petroclinoid fold connects between posterior clinoid and petrous apex and interclinoid fold between both the clinoids, and the oculomotor triangle is between these folds. The oculomotor nerve with its cuff will enter the roof to reach the lateral wall.

The oculomotor nerve, trochlear nerve, and ophthalmic branch of the trigeminal nerve (V1) course in the lateral wall of the cavernous sinus. The maxillary division of trigeminal nerve (V2) runs posteriorly along the lateral side and anteriorly along the floor of the sinus (**Fig. 8.22**). The abducent nerve enters the cavernous sinus through the dural foramen from the Dorello's canal and runs lateral to ICA.[6] The cavernous sinus triangles are spaces between the nerves in

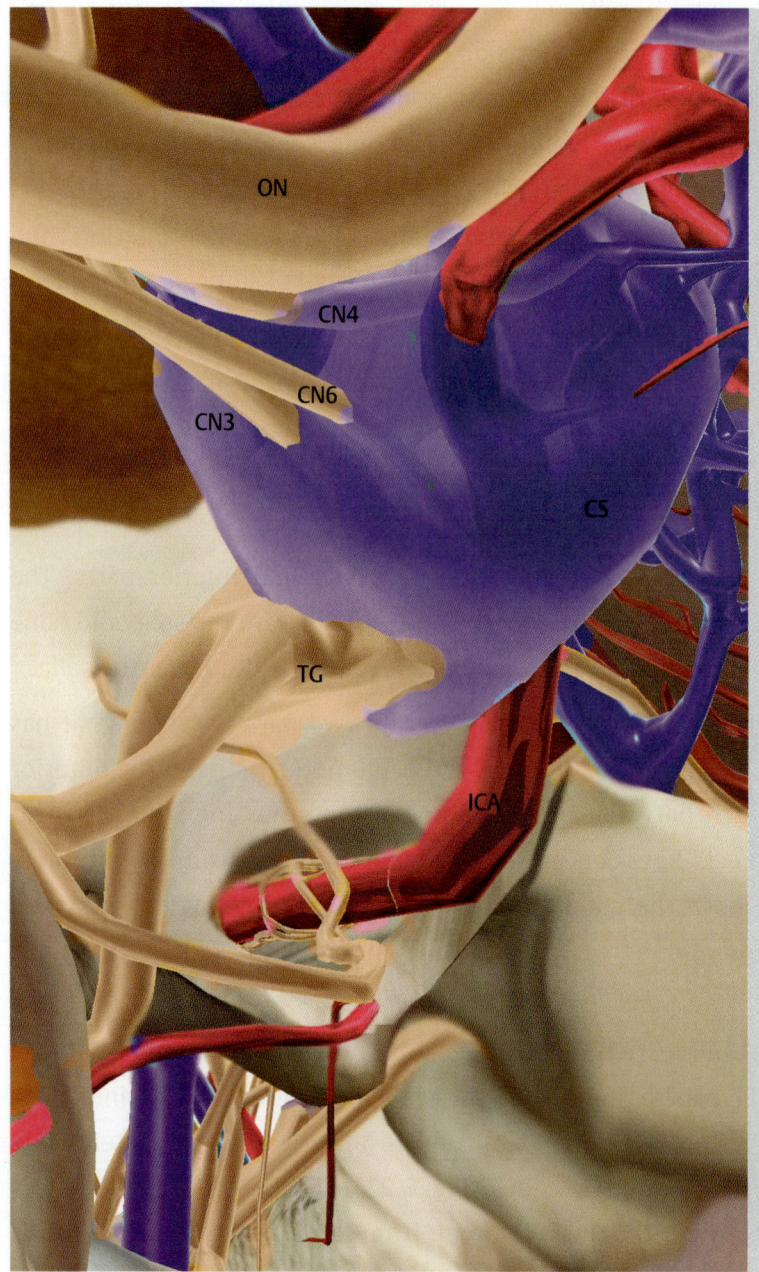

Fig. 8.22 Illustration showing contents of the coronal plane. ON, optic nerve; CN3, oculomotor nerve; CN4, trochlear nerve; CN6, abducent nerve; CS, cavernous sinus; TG, trigeminal ganglion; ICA, internal carotid artery.

the cavernous sinus which are supratrochlear, infratrochlear triangle (Parkinson's triangle), anteromedial, anterolateral, posterolateral, and posteromedial triangles (Kawase's triangle). The inferior border of cavernous sinus is present at the level of V2, so anterolateral, posterolateral, and posteromedial triangles are said to be middle fossa triangles (**Fig. 8.23**).

- Supratrochlear triangle—between the oculomotor and trochlear nerve
- Infratrochlear triangle—between the trochlear and V1 division of the trigeminal nerve
- Anteromedial triangle—between V1 and V2 divisions of trigeminal nerve.
- Anterolateral triangle—between V2 and V3 divisions of the trigeminal nerve
- Posterolateral triangle—between V3 and greater petrosal nerve
- Posteromedial triangle (Kawase's triangle)—between the greater petrosal nerve and trigeminal ganglion and superior petrosal sinus[6]

The cavernous internal carotid artery (ICA) gives two branches inside the cavernous sinus: the inferior cavernous sinus artery and meningohypophyseal trunk. This trunk will emerge on the medial compartment of the cavernous sinus and will give three branches: the tentorial artery, inferior hypophyseal artery, and dorsal meningeal artery.

Dissection

Dissection commences adopting a bi-nostril fourhanded approach with a 0-degree endoscope. A modified Denker's approach is performed, and the dissection of the PPF, as described earlier, is completed.

After the PPF is dissected, the SPA and DPA are clipped and the contents of PPF are dissected lateral from the underlying bone of the pterygoid wedge. Pterygoid wedge is the anterior junction of the medial and lateral pterygoid plates at their base. Pterygoid wedge is drilled from the V2 (maxillary division of the trigeminal nerve) superolaterally to the vidian canal inferomedially (**Fig. 8.24**). On removing

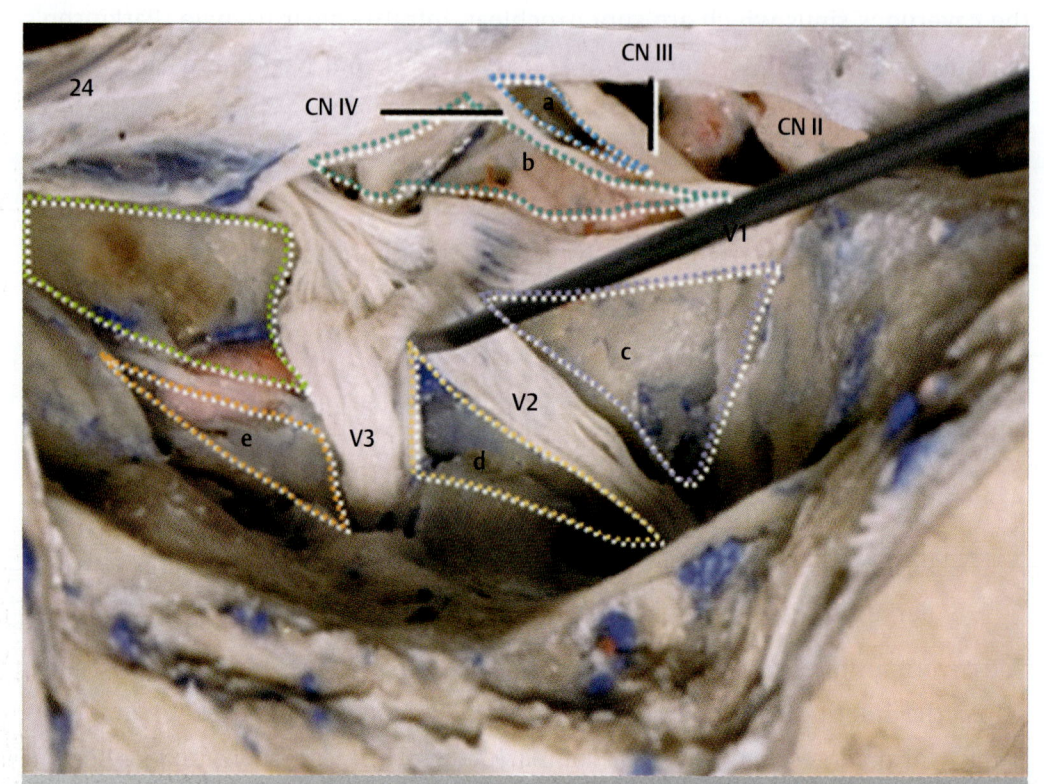

Fig. 8.23 The inner dural layer and the venous contents of the right cavernous sinus have been removed. The parasellar and middle fossa triangles are the spaces between the nerves and can be selectively opened to access specific areas of the cavernous sinus or surrounding structures. Removing the endosteal layer and the venous plexus in the middle fossa and parasellar area exposes the supratrochlear (a), infratrochlear (b) (or Parkinson's), anteromedial (c), anterolateral (d), posterolateral (e), and posteromedial (f) triangles. As the inferior border of the cavernous sinus is located at the level of the maxillary division and foramen rotundum, the anterolateral, posterolateral and posteromedial triangles are considered middle fossa triangles. The anterolateral triangle is located between the maxillary and mandibular divisions and contains the motor trigeminal root. The posterolateral triangle (e) is bordered anteriorly by the mandibular division, and medially by the greater petrosal nerve. The posteromedial or Kawase's triangle (f) is located medial to the greater petrosal nerve and is related to the trigeminal ganglion and superior petrosal sinus. CN: cranial nerve; V1: first division; V2: second division; V3: third division of trigeminal nerve. (Reproduced from Stamm A. Transnasal Endoscopic Skull Base and Brain Surgery. Tips and Pearls. ©2011, Thieme Publishers, New York.)

Endoscopic Approaches in Coronal Plane

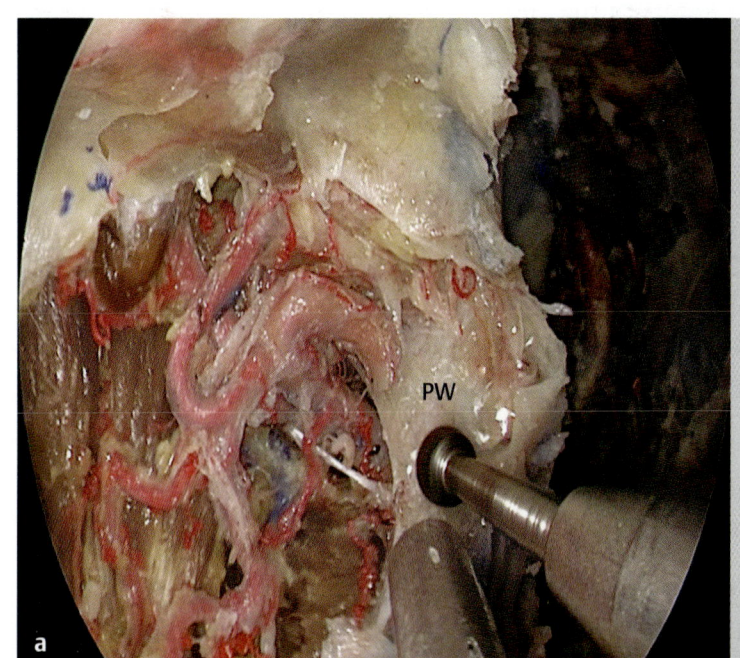

Fig. 8.24 Endoscopic image showing **(a)** drilling of the bone of the pterygoid wedge (PW). **(b)** Lateral recess (LR) of the sphenoid sinus exposed after drilling the PW. V2, maxillary nerve; VC, vidian canal.

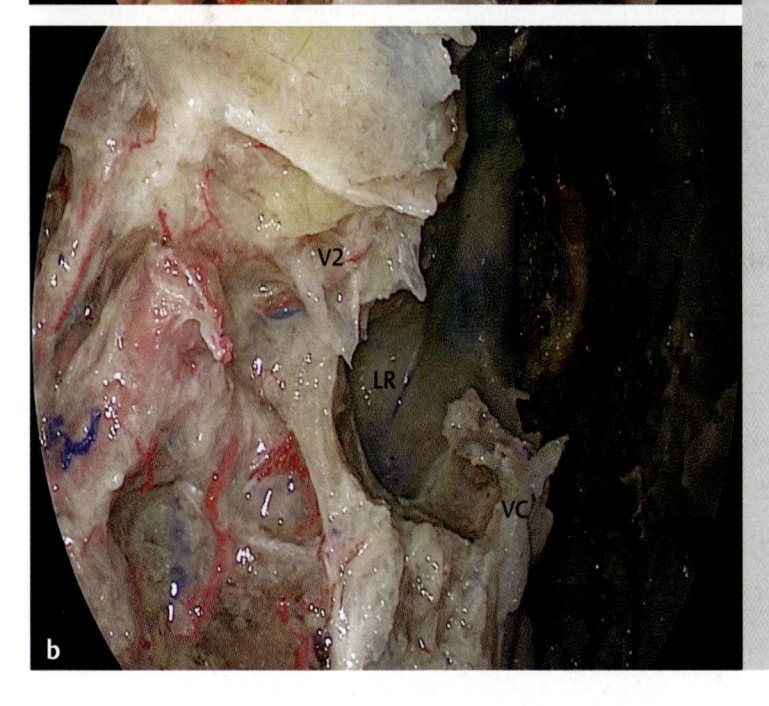

this bone, the dissection enters in the lateral recess of the sphenoid sinus. *The V2 and vidian canal are traced proximally to the Meckel's cave and ICA, respectively, and are the two most important landmarks in this dissection.*

The pterygoid canal, which is embedded in the floor of the sphenoid sinus, is now drilled along its inferior hemicircumference till anterior of the ICA canal (**Fig. 8.25**). The vidian artery, which is a content of the canal, is a branch of the ICA and is a fundamental landmark for identifying it as the ICA that lies in its superior margin. Once the ICA is identified at the level of anterior genu, a complete exposure of the paraclival and parasellar ICA is achieved (**Fig. 8.26**).

Now the V2 is traced proximally to locate the foramen rotundum, and drilling of the lateral wall of sphenoid sinus (**Fig. 8.27**) (maxillary strut) is further continued along the V2 until it pierces the middle fossa dura. The drilling continues laterally to the paraclival carotid artery to expose the middle fossa dura (**Fig. 8.28**) along the superior orbital fissure, mandibular nerve V3, and Meckel's cave (**Fig. 8.29**). This completes the extradural part of the approach to the Meckel's cave (**Fig. 8.30**).

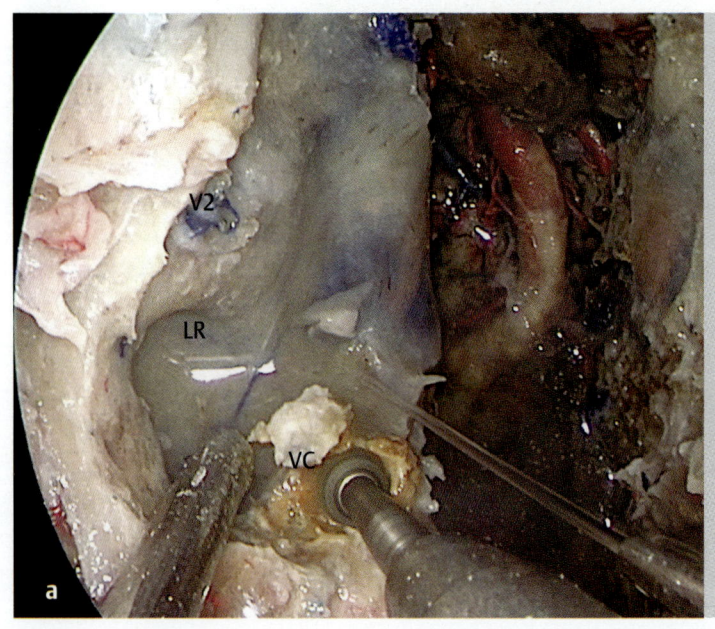

Fig. 8.25 (a) Endoscopic image showing drilling of the pterygoid canal along its inferior hemicircumference.

Endoscopic Approaches in Coronal Plane

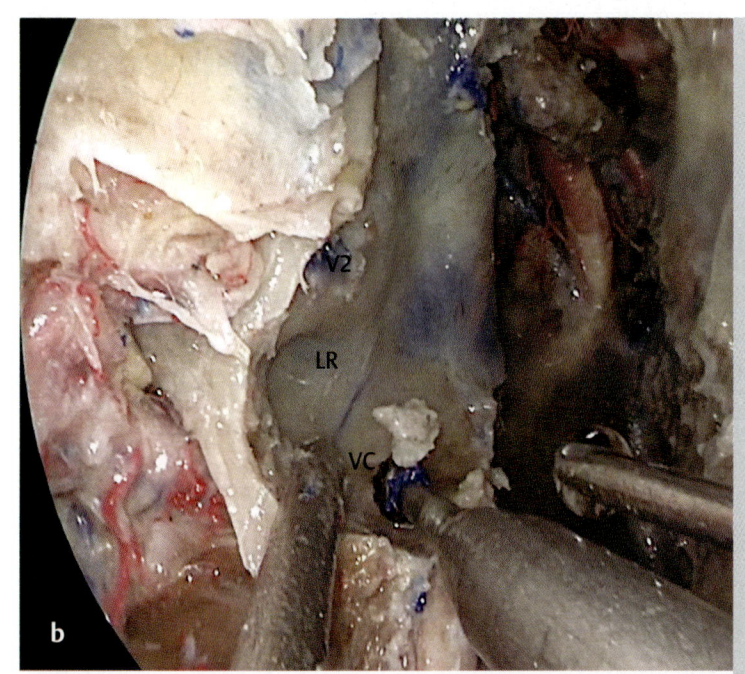

Fig. 8.25 (b) Drilling is continued up till the anterior genu of the paraclival internal carotid artery (PCICA) canal. **(c)** Vidian nerve (VN) in lateral relation to the PCICA. LR, lateral recess; V2, maxillary nerve; VC, vidian canal.

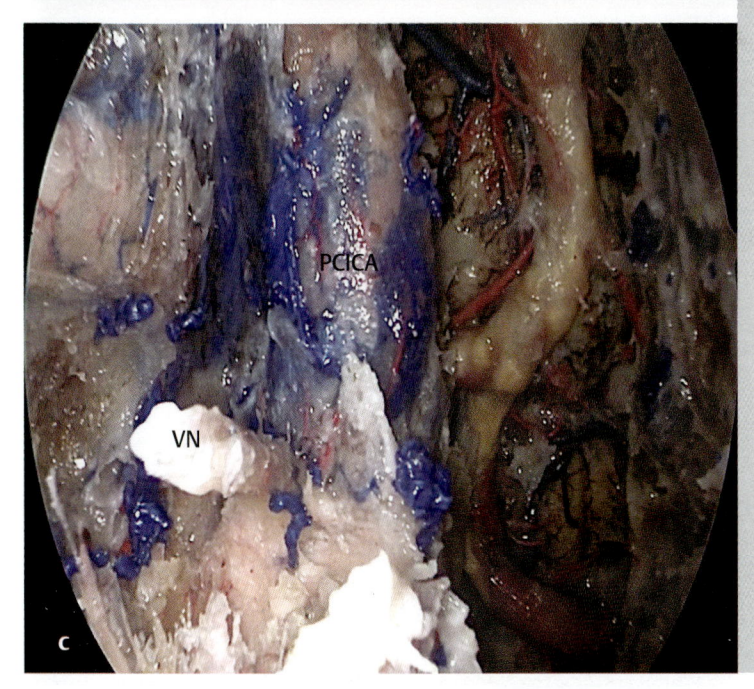

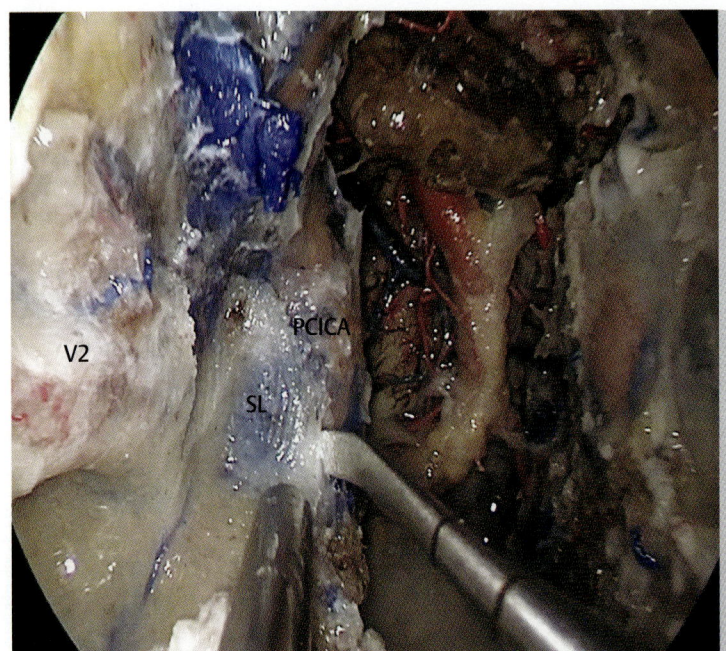

Fig. 8.26 Endoscopic image showing exposure of paraclival internal carotid artery (pcica). SL, lingula of sphenoid bone.

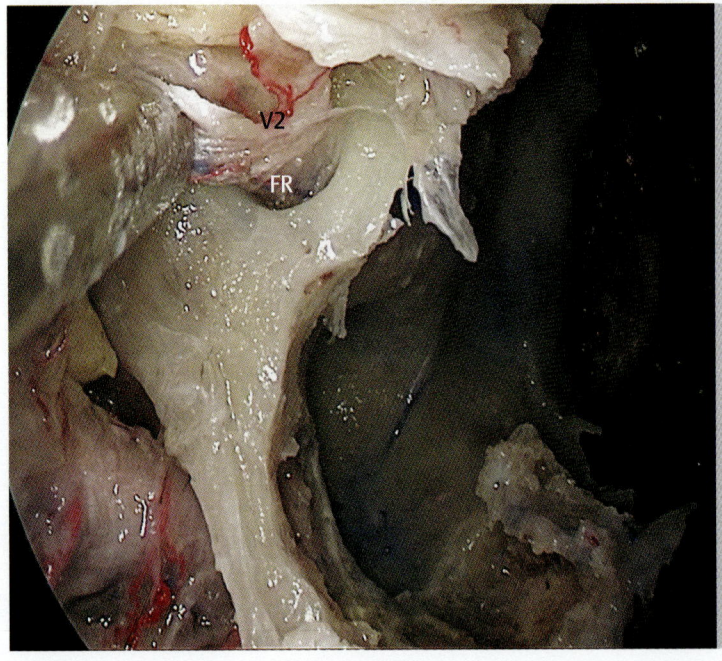

Fig. 8.27 Endoscopic image showing the maxillary nerve (V2) arising from the foramen rotundum (FR).

Endoscopic Approaches in Coronal Plane

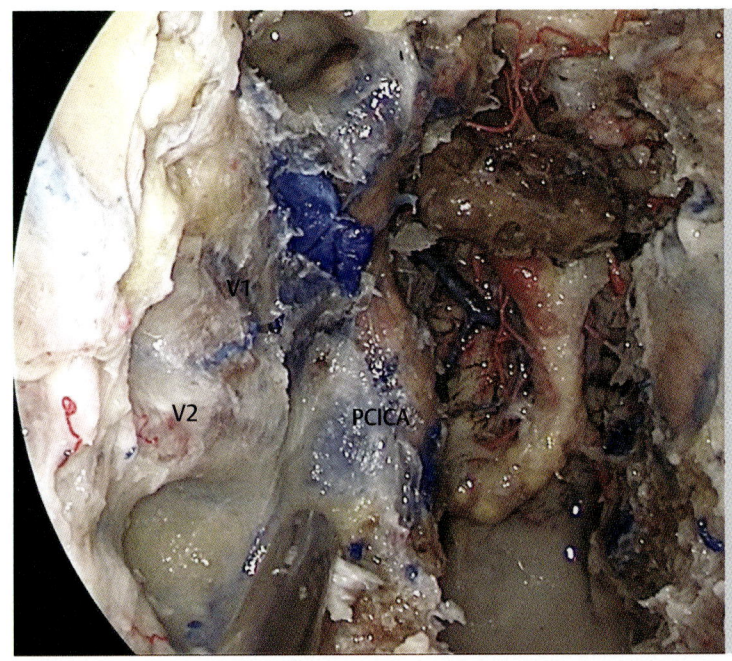

Fig. 8.28 Endoscopic image showing removal of bone over maxillary nerve (V2). PCICA, paraclival internal carotid artery; V1, ophthalmic nerve.

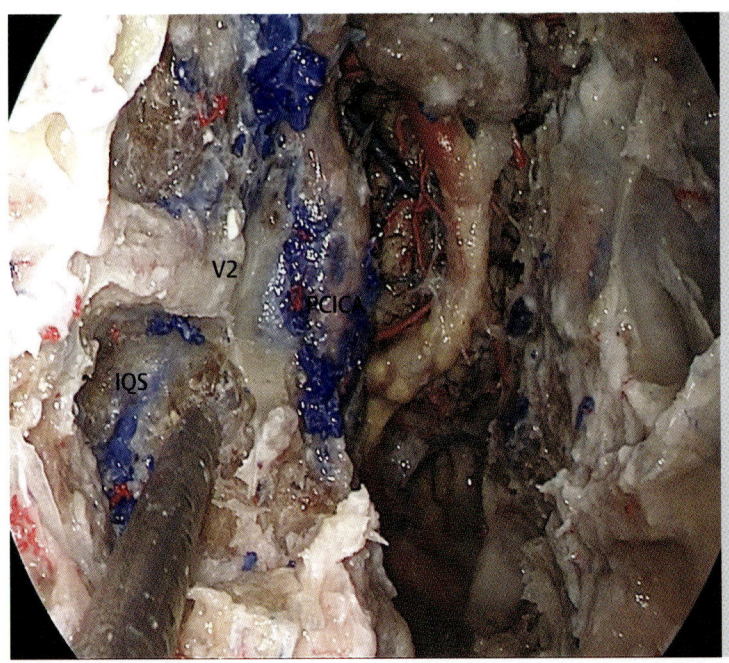

Fig. 8.29 Endoscopic image showing removal of lingual process of sphenoid below maxillary nerve (V2). IQS, inferior quadrangular space; PCICA, paraclival internal carotid artery.

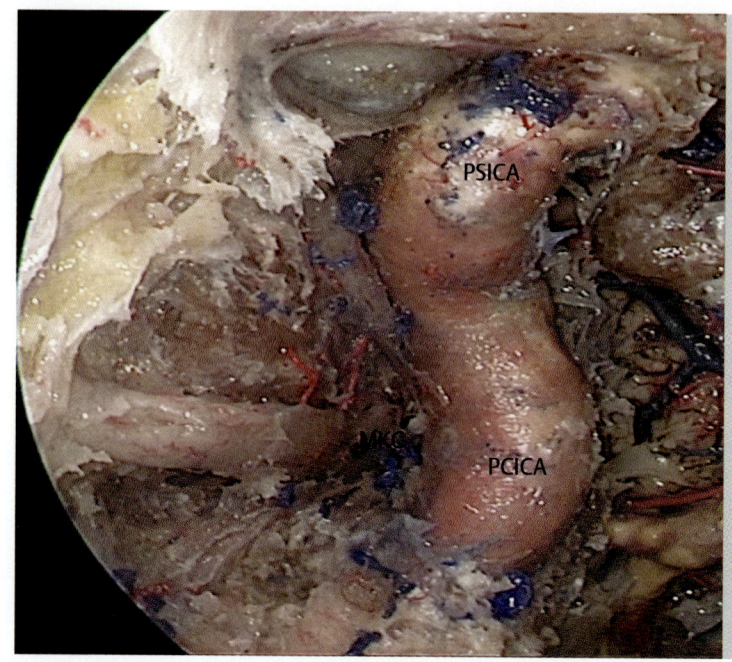

Fig. 8.30 Endoscopic image showing extra dural exposure for transpterygoid approach to Meckel's cave (MC). PCICA, paraclival internal carotid artery; PSICA, parasellar internal carotid artery.

The intradural part is accessed by opening the periosteum in a quadrangular space bounded by the horizontal petrous ICA inferiorly, vertical paraclival ICA medially, V2 laterally, and abducent nerve (cranial nerve [CN] VI) superiorly. The dissection is carried out inferior to the V2 to avoid injury to the CN VI that is in close relation to the ophthalmic division (V1). The trigeminal nerve is identified by dividing at the Meckel's cave.

Transpterygoid Approach to Superior Cavernous Sinus

The indications of this approach are rare, and the risk of this approach in absence of ophthalmoplegia should be duly weighed against the benefits of such a procedure. This approach is implemented in invasive secreting pituitary adenomas where a complete clearance is necessary.

Endoscopic Approaches in Coronal Plane

This approach is an extension of the suprapetrous approach to the inferior cavernous sinus, as described previously. A similar kind of exposure is obtained with the horizontal petrous, and the vertical paraclival ICA is exposed. Here, however, a larger middle fossa dura is exposed by drilling the bone from orbital apex anterosuperiorly to V2 anteroinferiorly, and from optic carotid recess posterosuperiorly to prominence of paraclival ICA posteroinferiorly. Additionally, the dural of the sella is incised to reconfirm the position of the medial ICA.

Once such an exposure is obtained and position of ICA is confirmed, the dura is incised very cautiously from medial to lateral direction until the CN VI and ICA are identified. Such an exposure is above the quadrangular space and CN VI (**Fig. 8.31**). This is an approach to the lateral and superior compartments of the cavernous sinus (**Fig. 8.32**). It is important to note, however, that in surgery, as contrast to a cadaveric dissection, the position of the intracavernous ICA is mapped with neuronavigation or with arterial Doppler.

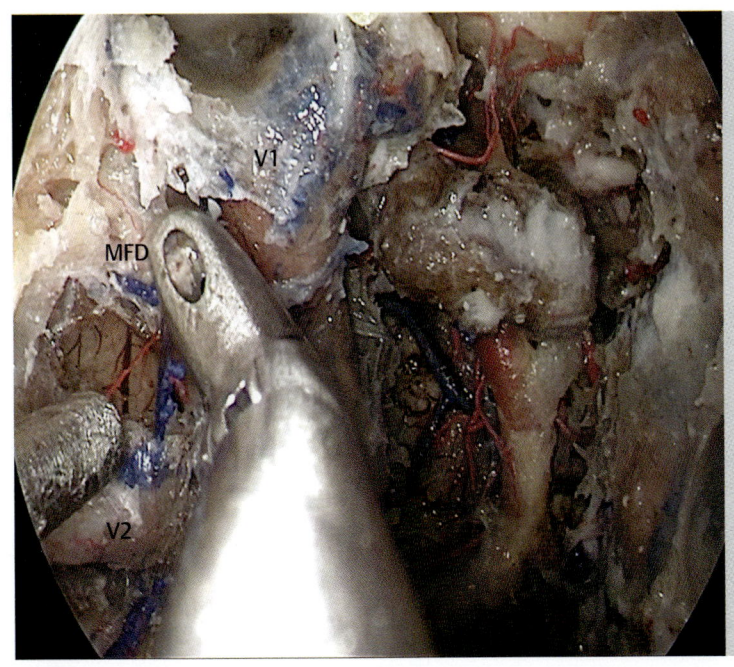

Fig. 8.31 Endoscopic image showing exposure in the upper quadrangular space. MFD, middle fossa dura in upper quadrangular space; V1, ophthalmic nerve; V2, maxillary nerve.

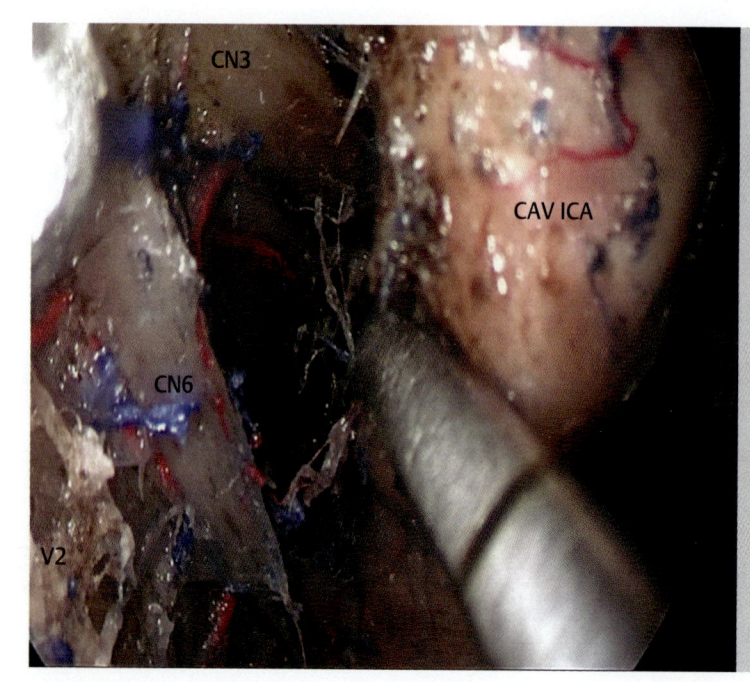

Fig. 8.32 Endoscopic image showing final exposure for transpterygoid approach to cavernous sinus. CN3, oculomotor nerve; CN4, trochlear nerve; CN6, abducent nerve; CAV ICA, cavernous internal cavernous artery; V2, maxillary nerve.

It is also important to understand that these approaches are preferred when the lesion itself creates corridor displacing the ICA medially and cranial nerves laterally. The lesions in the lateral cavernous sinus that do not displace ICA or cranial nerves are difficult to access by these approaches.

To approach the medial and posterosuperior compartments of the cavernous sinus, an endoscopic midline transsphenoidal approach is used. In this approach after a thorough trans-sellar exposure, the tumor is followed through the C-shaped curve of the intracavernous ICA from sella to the cavernous sinus using a cavernous sinus suction tip. This approach is elaborated in the chapter 7.

Posterior Coronal Approach

Infrapetrous Transpterygoid Approach

A similar transpterygoid access is gained, and the ICA is identified at the anterior genu by tracing the vidian canal proximally. Once ICA is identified, the nasopharyngeal soft tissue and median part of the ET are resected. The position of the parapharyngeal carotid artery is confirmed. And the bone inferior and medial to the anterior genu of the carotid artery is cautiously drilled to gain access to the petrous bone. Now curved suctions and irrigation can be used in surgery to extirpate lesion of the inferior or medial petrous like cholesterol granuloma or cholesteatoma.

This completes the description of the most commonly used endoscopic ventral skull base approaches in coronal plane.

Conclusion

The authors have detailed endoscopic endonasal approaches to various anatomical subunits along the three coronal planes. These trajectories can be used singly or in combination to gain complete access to lesions as well as to achieve neurovascular control. These can also be combined with external approaches for extensive lesions that are not accessible by endoscopic approaches alone.

A thorough knowledge of endoscopic anatomy and surgical skills gained over long hours of dissections facilitate an endoscopic skull base surgeon to deal with learning curve and achieve superior surgical outcomes.

References

1. Kassam AB, Gardner PA. Endoscopic approaches to the skull base. Prog Neurol Surg 2012;26:104–118

2. Karakaş P, Bozkir MG, Oguz O. Morphometric measurements from various reference points in the orbit of male Caucasians. Surg Radiol Anat 2003;24(6):358–362

3. Tsirbas A, Kazim M, Close L. Endoscopic approach to orbital apex lesions. Ophthal Plast Reconstr Surg 2005;21(4):271–275

4. Upadhyay S, Dolci RLL, Buohliqah L, et al. Effect of incremental endoscopic maxillectomy on surgical exposure of the pterygopalatine and infratemporal fossae. J Neurol Surg B Skull Base 2016;77(1):66–74

5. Vescan AD, Snyderman CH, Carrau RL, et al. Vidian canal: analysis and relationship to the internal carotid artery. Laryngoscope 2007;117(8):1338–1342

6. Chung BS, Ahn YH, Park JS. Ten triangles around cavernous sinus for surgical approach, described by schematic diagram and three dimensional models with the sectioned images. J Korean Med Sci 2016;31(9):1455–1463

Index

Note: Page numbers followed by *f* and *t* indicate figures and tables, respectively.

A
Adrenaline lint, 30, 30*f*
Agger nasi, 54*f*, 109
    after removal of uncinate vertical limb, 54, 54*f*
    anterior and medial wall removal of, 55*f*
    uncapping, 54*f*
Aircraft technique, 38–39
Alar elasticity, 20, 20*f*
Angled scopes
    30-degree telescope, 28, 28*f*
    70-degree telescope, 28, 28*f*
Anterior coronal plane, anatomical subunits in, 157
Anterior coronal plane, endoscopic approaches in
    optic nerve decompression, 163–165
    orbital decompression, 158–159
Anterior ethmoidal fovea, 51
Anterior ethmoid cells, dissection of, 56–58, 58*f*
Anterior skull base anatomy, 75

B
Backbiting forceps, 44, 45*f*
Bi-nostril technique, 76
Blakesley forceps, 47
Bulla, 56

C
Cadaveric dissections, 76
    endonasal vascularized flaps, 86, 86*t*
    instrumentation for, 9
    skull base, 75
Camera
    and light source cables, position of, 20, 20*f*
    tilt, 32, 32*f*
Cavernous sinus anatomy, 181, 182*f*
Cold steel instruments, 9, 12*f*
Computed tomography (CT), 75
Constant distance principle, 25, 25*f*, 26*f*, 27*f*
Crossover phenomenon, 23, 23*f*

D
Denker's procedure, 167–169, 169*f*
Descending palatine artery (DPA), 176*f*

E
Endonasal endoscopic approaches, advantages of, 75
Endonasal endoscopic corridor, 3
Endonasal endoscopic surgery, 3
    challenges associated with, 4
Endonasal endoscopy, ergonomics in, 4
Endonasal skull-base surgery, 3
Endonasal vascularized flaps, 86, 86*t*
Endoscope, holding of, 19, 19*f*
Endoscopic approaches in sagittal plane
    endoscopic transnasal craniectomy approach
        applications, 116
        division of falx, 118, 120*f*
        drilling of fovea, 116, 118*f*
        frontopolar and frontorbital vessels, 118, 121*f*
        incising of dura, 118, 119*f*
        retraction of ethmoidal roof, 118, 119*f*
        transection of olfactory tract, 118, 121*f*
    endoscopic transnasal transsphenoidal approaches
        nasal phase, 128–132, 130*f*, 132*f*
    transclival approach
        lower clivus dissection, 147, 150, 150*f*
        mid-clival dissection, 147, 148*f*
        reconstruction, 150, 152, 153*f*
        upper clivus dissection, 142–146, 144*f*, 145*f*, 146*f*
    transfrontal approach, 107
        applications, 107
        bi-nostril four-handed approach, 112
        0-degree endoscope, 110
        drilling, 113, 114*f*, 115*f*
        frontal "T," 113, 115*f*
        initial entry into frontal sinus, 113, 114*f*
        inverted U-shaped incision, 110, 113*f*
        mucosa removal, 110, 111*f*

Index

superior septectomy, 110, 112f
two-handed uni-nostril approach, 110
transplanum approach, 136–140, 139f, 140, 140f
trans-sellar approach, 125f, 133–135
transtuberculum approach, 136, 137f
Endoscopic approaches in ventral skull base surgery, 157
  anterior coronal plane
    optic nerve decompression, 163–165
    orbital decompression, 158–159
  middle coronal plane, 166–192
    approach to infratemporal fossa, 177–178
    Denker's procedure, 167–169
    endoscopic medial maxillectomy, 166–167
    posterior coronal approach, 193
    suprapetrous transpterygoid approach, 178–190
    transpterygoid approach, 190–192
    transpterygoid approach to pterygopalatine fossa, 170–177
Endoscopic camera system, 9, 10f, 11f
Endoscopic dacryocystorhinostomy, 66–71
  frontal process of maxilla, 67, 69f
  incision marking, 67, 67f
  inferiorly based mucosal flap, 67, 69f
    repositioned, 68, 71f
  lacrimal sac
    endosteal layer of, 68, 70f
    and nasolacrimal duct, 69f
Endoscopic instruments, 9
Endoscopic medial maxillectomy, 157, 166–167
Endoscopic sinus surgery
  functional, 3
  history of, 3
Endoscopic sinus surgery, basic steps of
  adrenaline lint, 30, 30f
  angled scopes
    30-degree telescope, 28, 28f
    70-degree telescope, 28, 28f
  camera tilt, 32, 32f
  constant distance principle, 25, 25f, 26f, 27f
  crossover phenomenon, 23, 23f
  endoscopic view of instrument tip, 24, 24f
  hemostatic measures, 29
  holding of endoscope, 19, 19f
  instrument below telescope, 29
  instrument introduction along floor, 23, 23f
  introduction of scope, 20, 20f
  middle turbinate manipulation, 31, 31f
  panoramic view, 29
  patient position
    extended position, 17, 19f
    flexed position, 17, 18f
    neutral position, 17, 18f
  position of camera and light source cables, 20, 20f
  semilunar sign, 21, 21f
Endoscopic skull base surgery, 76
  definition, 9
  instrumentation for, 9
  prerequisite for, 9
Endoscopic transnasal craniectomy approach
  applications, 116
  division of falx, 118, 120f
  drilling of fovea, 116, 118f
  frontopolar and frontorbital vessels, 118, 121f
  incising of dura, 118, 119f
  retraction of ethmoidal roof, 118, 119f
  transection of olfactory tract, 118, 121f
Endoscopic transnasal transsphenoidal approaches, 122, 130f, 132f
Ethmoidal bulla, 109
Ethmoidal neurovascular bundle
  anterior, 65
  posterior, 64
Ethmoidal notch, 110
Ethmoid pneumatization, 109
Extra dural exposure, 190f

F

Falx cerebri, 110
Fovea drilling, 118f
Frontal bone, cranial surface of, 109
Frontal bulla, 109
Frontal cells, 52
Frontal crest, 110
Frontal ostium, 109
Frontal recess
  boundaries of, 52
  frontal sinus visualized through, 55f
Frontal recess dissection
  intact bulla technique, 53
  medial drainage, 53
Frontal sinus
  anterior wall, 108
  drainage pathways for, 37
  drilling of IFS connecting, 117f

Index

inferior wall, 109
medial wall, 108
ostium, 109
posterior wall, 108
transillumination of, 53
visualized through frontal recess, 55f
Frontal sinus recess
　boundaries of, 51
　noninflammatory pathologies, 51
　supra-agger/frontal/frontoethmoidal cells, 52
　suprabullar cell, 52
　supraorbital ethmoidal cell, 52
Frontoethmoidal cells, 52
Frontonasal duct, 109
Functional endoscopic sinus surgery (FESS), 10
　basic operative etiquettes, 77
　cadaver dissections for, 37–38
　indications for, 37
　instruments dedicated for, 12f
　popularity, 37

H

Hadad–Bassagasteguy flap (HBF), 86–90
　incisions, 88, 89f
　indicated in CSF leaks, 88
　lateralization of inferior turbinate, 88
　nasal septum, 86
　placement for anterior skull base defect, 90, 90f
　sphenopalatine artery, 86, 87f
Hemostatic measures, 29
High-speed neurodrill systems, 9–10, 13f

I

Inferior turbinate flap, 91–95
　incision, 91, 92f
　medialized, 91
　placement of, 91, 95f
　raising, 91, 94f
Inferior turbinate resection, 167f
Inflammatory sinus pathology, 37
Infrapetrous transpterygoid approach, 193
Infratemporal fossa
　approach to, 177–178
　complete exposure of, 179f
　contents of, 179f
Instrumentation
　definition, 9
　importance, 9
Internal maxillary artery, 176f

L

Lacrimal sac, 66
Lamina papyracea, 109, 160, 161f
Lateral optic recess, 123
Lateral periosteal flap elevation, 168f
Lateral recess, 123
Lateral sphenoidal wall, 124f
Lingual process removal, 189f

M

Mandibular nerve, 179f
Maxillary antrum, 170f
Maxillary nerve, 187f
Maxillary sinuses, drainage pathways for, 37
Meckel's cave, 178
Medial and lateral optic carotid recess, 123f
Medial drainage, 53
Medial optic carotic recess, 123
Messerklinger technique, 37
Microdebrider, 14f, 47
Middle coronal plane, endoscopic approaches in, 166–192
　approach to infratemporal fossa, 177–178
　Denker's procedure, 167–169
　endoscopic medial maxillectomy, 166–167
　posterior coronal approach, 193
　suprapetrous transpterygoid approach, 178–190
　transpterygoid approach, 190–192
　transpterygoid approach to pterygopalatine fossa, 170–177
Middle meatal antrostomy
　definition, 47
　guidelines for, 49
　technique, 47–50, 48f, 50f
Middle turbinate (MT), 39
Middle turbinate flap, 96–97, 97f
　indications, 96
　manipulation, 31, 31f
Mucosal flap, 66

N

Nasal endoscopy, 3, 38–39
Nasal mucosa, vascularized, 85
Nasofrontal beak, 110

O

Optic nerve decompression, 163–165
Orbital apex, transorbital approach to, 162f
Orbital decompression, 158–159

Index

Orbital fat, removal of, 162f
Orbit, removal of floor of, 161f
Osteomeatal complex (OMC), 37

P

Paraclival internal carotid artery (PCICA), 187f
Partial endoscopic maxillectomy, 157
Patient position
    extended position, 17, 19f
    flexed position, 17, 18f
    neutral position, 17, 18f
Pedicled flaps, 86
Pericranial flap, 98–102
    harvested, 98, 101f
    incision, 98, 99f, 100f
    supraorbital and supratrochlear artery, 98
Periosteum, 175f
Pneumatization of frontal bone, 51
Posterior coronal approach, 193
Posterior ethmoid
    boundaries, 59
    dissection, 59–60, 60f
Posterior lateral nasal artery, 91
Posterior wall of maxillary sinus (PWMS), 171f
Primary inflammatory process, 37
Pterygoid canal drilling, 186f
Pterygoid recess, 124
Pterygoid wedge (PW), 183, 185f
Pterygopalatine fossa
    dissection of, 173–177
    transpterygoid approach to, 170–177
Pterygopalatine fossa (PPF)
    anatomy, 172–173
    endoscopic approach to, 170–177

S

Semilunar sign, 21, 21f
Shaver system, 10, 14f
Sinus physiology, functional restoration of, 37
Skull-base reconstruction
    goals of, 85
    resource for, 85–86
Skull base training, 75
Sphenoethmoidal recess, 38
Sphenoid osteum, 56
Sphenoid sinus
    anatomy of, 122–126
    anterior extension of, 124
    anterior wall of, 124
    carotid prominence in, 125
    dissection, 61–65
        skull base, 64f
        structures, 61, 63f
        widened frontal recess, 65f
    extensive pneumatization of, 123
    floor of, 125
    lateral recess, 185f
    ostium of, 124
    posterior wall of, 125
    roof of, 125
    routes to approach, 61
    sphenopalatine artery, 126
Sphenopalatine artery (SPA), 86, 87f, 174f, 176f
Superior alveolar artery, 176f
Supra-agger cells, 52
Suprabullar cell, 52
Supraoptic recess, 123
Supraorbital and supratrochlear artery, 98
Supraorbital ethmoidal cell, 52
Suprapetrous transpterygoid approach, 178–190

T

Tactile feedback, 9
Transclival approach
    lower clivus dissection, 147, 150, 150f
    mid-clival dissection, 147, 148f, 149f
    reconstruction, 150, 152, 153f
    upper clivus dissection, 142–146, 144f, 145f, 146f
Transcribriform approach, 107
Transfrontal approach, 107
    applications, 107
    bi-nostril four-handed approach, 112
    0-degree endoscope, 110
    drilling, 113, 114f, 115f
    frontal "T," 113, 115f
    initial entry into frontal sinus, 113, 114f
    inverted U-shaped incision, 110, 113f
    mucosa removal, 110, 111f
    superior septectomy, 110, 112f
    two-handed uni-nostril approach, 110
Transillumination of frontal sinus, 53
Transplanum approach, 136–140, 139f, 140, 140f
Transpterygoid approach, 190–192
    infrapetrous, 193
    to pterygopalatine fossa, 170–177
    to superior cavernous sinus, 190–192
    suprapetrous, 178–190

Index

Trans-sellar approach, 125f, 133–135
Transsphenoidal approach, 125
Transtuberculum approach, 136, 137f

U
Uncinate bone, horizontal portion of, 49
"Uncinate Flap" technique, 47
Uncinate, horizontal limb of
    removal of, 46f
    submucosal dissection of, 45f
Uncinate process, 109
Uncinectomy
    dissection, 42–43, 42f, 43f
    technique, 44, 45f, 46f
    uncinate process, 39–41, 41f
    using backbiting forceps, 45f

V
Vascularized flaps, endonasal, 86, 86t
Vascularized pedicled flaps, dissection of
    demand for, 102
    Hadad–Bassagasteguy flap (HBF), 86–90
        incisions, 88, 89f
        indicated in CSF leaks, 88
        lateralization of inferior turbinate, 88
        nasal septum, 86
        placement for anterior skull base defect, 88, 90f
        sphenopalatine artery, 86, 87f
    inferior turbinate flap, 91–95
        incision, 91, 92f
        medialized, 91
        placement of, 91, 95f
        raising, 91, 94f
    middle turbinate flap, 96–97, 97f
        indications, 96
    pericranial flap, 98–102
        harvested, 98, 101f
        incision, 98, 99f, 100f
        supraorbital and supratrochlear artery, 98
Ventral skull base, 75
Ventral skull base instrumentation
    cold steel instruments, 9, 12f
    endoscopes used in, 11f
    endoscopic camera system, 9, 10f, 11f
    high-speed neurodrill systems, 9–10, 13f
    instruments for dissection, 10f, 11f, 12f, 13f, 14f
    shaver system, 10, 14f
Ventral skull base (VSB) surgery, 3–4
    advancement in, 76
    basic operative etiquettes, 77
    bimanual dissection, 78
    bi-nostril four-handed approach, 77–78, 80f
    cadaveric dissections, 81, 81f
    coordinated effort, 80
    endoscope and suction cannula, position of, 79, 79f
    endoscopic approaches in (*See* Endoscopic approaches in ventral skull base surgery)
    instruments dedicated for, 12f
    instruments for, 80
    mastering, 75
    posterior septectomy, 78, 78f
    preoperative planning and reconstruction, 77
    skill acquisition, 81
    wide exposure, 77
Vidian nerve (VN), 187f